P9-DWZ-614

WHO Technical Report Series
865

CONTROL OF
HEREDITARY DISEASES

Report of a
WHO Scientific Group

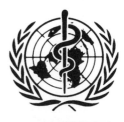

World Health Organization

Geneva 1996

)ata

Hereditary Diseases (1993 : Geneva, Switzerland)
of a WHO scientific group.

(WHO technical report series ; 865)

1. Hereditary diseases – prevention and control
2. Genetics, Medical   3. Gene therapy   4. Human genome project
I. Title II. Series

ISBN 92 4 120865 1   (NLM Classification: QZ 50)
ISSN 0512-3054

The World Health Organization welcomes requests for permission to reproduce or translate its publications, in part or in full. Applications and enquiries should be addressed to the Office of Publications, World Health Organization, Geneva, Switzerland, which will be glad to provide the latest information on any changes made to the text, plans for new editions, and reprints and translations already available.

© World Health Organization 1996

Printed in Switzerland
95/10781 – Benteli – 7000

Contents

WHO Scientific Group on the Control of Hereditary Diseases

Geneva, 23–25 November 1993

Members

Professor K. Berg, Chairman, Institute of Medical Genetics, University of Oslo, Ulleval University Hospital, Oslo, Norway (*Chairman*)

Professor B. Brambati, First Obstetric Clinic, Faculty of Medicine, Milan University, Milan, Italy

Professor N. Fujiki, Department of Internal Medicine and Medical Genetics, Fukui Medical School, Fukui, Japan

Professor E. K. Ginter, Director, Institute of Medical Genetics, Russian Academy of Medical Sciences, Moscow, Russian Federation

Professor B. M. Knoppers, Faculty of Law, University of Montreal, Montreal, Quebec, Canada

Professor B. Modell, Perinatal Centre, Department of Obstetrics and Gynaecology, University College and Middlesex School of Medicine, London, England (*Rapporteur*)

Professor I. C. Verma, Genetics Unit, Department of Pediatrics, All India Institute of Medical Sciences, New Delhi, India (*Vice-Chairman*)

Professor R. Williamson, Department of Biochemistry and Molecular Genetics, St Mary's Hospital Medical School, Imperial College, London, England

Representatives of other organizations

Council for International Organizations of Medical Sciences (CIOMS)
Dr Z. Bankowski, Secretary-General, CIOMS, Geneva, Switzerland

International Clearinghouse for Birth Defects Monitoring Systems (ICBDMS)
Professor E. Castilla, Vice-Chairperson, ICBDMS, Department of Genetics, Oswaldo Cruz Institute, Rio de Janeiro, Brazil

International Cystic Fibrosis (Mucoviscidosis) Association (ICF(M)A)
Professor J. A. Dodge, Chairman, Scientific Medical Advisory Council, ICF(M)A, Nuffield Department of Child Health, Institute of Clinical Science, Queen's University, Belfast, Northern Ireland
Mrs L. Heidet, ICF(M)A/WHO Liaison Officer, Geneva, Switzerland
Mr M. Weibel, President, ICF(M)A, Uetendorf, Switzerland

International Neurofibromatosis Association (INFA)
Mr P. R. W. Bellermann, Chairman, INFA, New York, NY, USA

World Federation of Hemophilia (WFH)
Professor P. M. Mannucci, Medical Vice-President, WFH, A. Bianchi Bonomi Haemophilia and Thrombosis Centre, Milan, Italy

Secretariat

Dr V. Boulyjenkov, Responsible Officer, Hereditary Diseases Programme, Division of Noncommunicable Diseases, WHO, Geneva, Switzerland (*Secretary*)

Dr E. N. Chigan, Director, Division of Noncommunicable Diseases, WHO, Geneva, Switzerland

Dr N. P. Napalkov, Assistant Director-General, WHO, Geneva, Switzerland

1. Introduction

The WHO Scientific Group on the Control of Hereditary Diseases met in Geneva from 23 to 25 November 1993 to review present applications of genetic knowledge and the future potential of that knowledge for improving human health. The meeting was opened by Dr N. P. Napalkov, Assistant Director-General, who welcomed participants on behalf of the Director-General, and said that developments in molecular biology were rapidly increasing the possibilities for avoiding or treating common conditions with a genetic predisposition, as well as classical genetic disorders. These developments not only had profound implications for human health, but also raised important social, ethical and legal issues.

Although the limits of intelligence, physical ability and longevity are genetically determined, environmental and external influences such as infections, malnutrition and war have hitherto been the main determinants of health and survival. Now, however, with increased control of the environment, genetic make-up is becoming a progressively more important determinant of the health of the individual. In developed countries, genetic disorders are responsible for a large proportion of infant mortality and childhood disability, and genetic predisposition may lead to the premature onset of common disorders of adult life such as diabetes, cancer, hypertension, coronary heart disease and dementia.

Until the 1970s, the approaches available for investigating the genetic contribution to disease were limited to family history, physical examination and conventional biochemical tests. Since then, the development of methods for handling, analysing and synthesizing DNA sequences has created biological tools for studying the basis of life itself, and, ultimately, for manipulating it.

Molecular biology now attracts many able researchers and much government and industrial interest, and research on human DNA is being coordinated internationally. The Human Genome Project is an international venture that aims, through systematic analysis, to achieve a complete picture of the sequence of human DNA. Although this objective is principally scientific, the information obtained will affect medical practice at many levels. Some of the new techniques for handling DNA are very simple, and are therefore likely to be applied universally; genetic approaches will help combat some of the commonest health problems of developing countries, including infectious disease.

The main medical application of DNA technology at present is in the diagnosis of genetic disorders, together with some common noncommunicable and infectious diseases; however, genes are being identified at an unprecedented rate, and the scope of genetic diagnosis and counselling is expanding rapidly as a result. Genetic contributions to common disorders are also beginning to be understood, and in the future it may be possible to treat or prevent premature disease by identifying

1

susceptible individuals, who can then be advised on lifestyle or provided with conventional or gene therapy.

Genetic approaches are thus set to become an integral part of many aspects of medical practice, and it is important for health workers to have a basic understanding of medical genetics in order to keep abreast of new developments. Unfortunately, most health professionals now in practice have been taught very little about medical genetics, and this is a serious problem that could limit the appropriate application of these new developments.

The task of the Scientific Group was therefore: (1) to review the place of genetics in modern medicine; (2) to summarize current practical applications of genetic knowledge in the diagnosis, treatment and prevention of disease; (3) to consider the likely immediate future impact of human genome research; (4) to help medical decision-makers to keep pace with these developments; and (5) to give guidance on the organization of genetic services.

The terms "abortion" and "termination of pregnancy" used in the text of this report are intended to mean "interruption of pregnancy following the detection of fetal abnormality". References to the procedure as a choice available to individuals and couples following a prenatal diagnosis assume that this is not prohibited by law in the country concerned. In this respect, WHO refers to the United Nations Report of the International Conference on Population and Development (Cairo, 5-13 September 1994) which states (para 8.25): "In no case should abortion be promoted as a method of family planning... Women who have unwanted pregnancies should have ready access to reliable information and compassionate counselling. Any measures or changes related to abortion within the health system can only be determined at the national or local level according to the national legislative process."

2. The human genome

2.1 The concept of the human genome

Figure 1 shows the double-helical molecular structure of DNA. Despite its complex role as the basis of life, DNA is a relatively simple molecule including only four bases – adenine, cytosine, guanine and thymine. Its two strands are held together by hydrogen bonds formed between these bases: adenine (A) can pair only with thymine (T) (by means of two hydrogen bonds) and cytosine (C) can pair only with guanine (G) (by means of three hydrogen bonds). Thus the two strands determine each other's base sequence, i.e. are complementary. When DNA replicates, the strands separate and DNA polymerase lays down a new complementary sequence on each strand, so that the sequence of bases is preserved at each cell division.

Figure 1
Structure of DNA

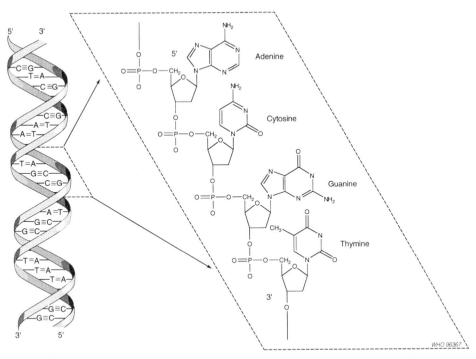

DNA consists of two strands of nucleotide bases strung along a sugar–phosphate "backbone" and twisted around each other in a double helix with the bases facing inwards. The four bases are adenine (A), thymine (T), cytosine (C) and guanine (G). The base sequence is the most important feature of DNA.

Genes are sections of DNA that code for, or direct the formation of, proteins (or RNA). Only one of the DNA strands is the coding or sense strand; the other – the antisense strand – is needed to maintain the stability and reproducibility of the molecule. In a coding sequence, each "triplet", or set of three bases, codes for one of 20 amino acids. The DNA sequence is translated by RNA into protein products. When a gene is "switched on", the double helix opens, and the enzyme RNA polymerase copies the coding sequence to make messenger RNA (mRNA). Then mRNA moves into the cytoplasm where it is decoded and translated into protein by the protein synthesis mechanism.

Most human DNA is contained in the 23 pairs of chromosomes in the cell nucleus (Fig. 2). Each chromosome consists of a single DNA molecule associated with proteins. DNA is not confined to the nucleus, however; mitochondria also have an independent and characteristic DNA complement, inherited only through the mother.

Different patterns of genes are "switched on" in each cell type. All cells contain proteins for cell life-support systems and for growth and division, plus structural proteins and enzymes characteristic of the tissue

3

Figure 2
Standard diagram of human chromosomes

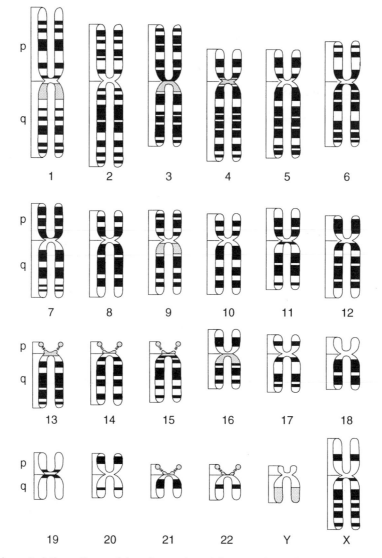

The characteristic pattern of bands produced by certain stains allows recognition of individual chromosomes. The nucleus of every human cell contains 23 pairs of chromosomes; one of each pair is inherited from the father and the other from the mother. One pair consists of the sex chromosomes (XX in females, XY in males); the other 22 pairs are referred to as autosomes. In the nucleus of a functioning cell, the chromosomes are extended and entwined; at cell division, they replicate and "condense" (i.e. become very tightly coiled), and two complete chromosome sets then separate in an orderly way into the two daughter cells. Chromosomes are easiest to observe microscopically when they are condensed during cell division, and hence are usually seen in duplexes (as here). When gametes are formed, spermatogonia and oogonia undergo a more complex division (meiosis), which yields gametes each containing a set of 23 chromosomes (22 autosomes and one sex chromosome). At fertilization, two gametes fuse to form a zygote with 46 chromosomes and the potential for embryonic development.

concerned. Embryonic development depends on the orderly switching on and off of sets of genes. Some code for specific embryonic proteins that do not appear in the adult, and others (proto-oncogenes) for growth-promoting factors. The latter are particularly important: their inappropriate activation as a consequence of somatic mutations can lead to cancer in later life.

There are probably about 80000–100000 genes, which are widely separated on the DNA strands (Fig. 3). Genes are themselves divided into coding sections ("exons") and intervening non-coding sections ("introns") (Fig. 4). The DNA between the genes contains structural sequences (responsible for the anatomy and behaviour of the chromosomes and for interaction with specific structural proteins) and controlling sequences (involved in switching genes on and off). In addition, about 30% of human DNA is composed of several kinds of variable-length repeating sequences.

A mutation is a spontaneous change in the sequence or the complement of DNA. There are two broad groups of mutations, namely *chromosomal abnormalities*, which are changes in chromosome number or arrangement, and *point mutations,* which are changes in the sequence of DNA bases. Mutation is an intrinsic property of DNA, and is the basis of evolution and of individual variation, but it can also give rise to genetic diseases and disorders.

Point mutations arise in only one of a pair of genes. When a single altered gene is sufficient to cause evident change, the mutation is termed dominant; if the presence of the remaining, unmutated gene prevents such change, the mutation is recessive. Many new mutations are lost from the population soon after they arise, either because they cause fatal disease or as a consequence of random events. Others become common because: the individual in whom the mutation arose leaves many descendants; the mutation confers a selective advantage on carriers (e.g. carriers of haemoglobin disorders and glucose-6-phosphate dehydrogenase (G6PD) deficiency are protected against malaria); or the mutation, though neutral, is closely associated with a gene that becomes common for one of the above reasons.

Figure 3
Chromosomal location (11p) and organization of the human β-globin gene cluster

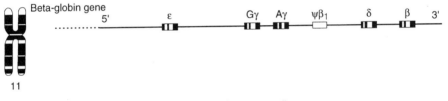

Genes are widely separated from each other by non-coding sequences.

Figure 4
Diagrammatic representation of the β-globin gene

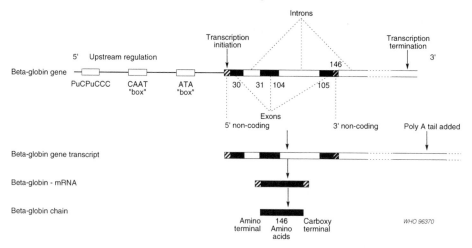

Genes are made up of a number of coding sequences (exons) separated by non-coding sequences (introns). They differ considerably in size; for example, the relatively small β-globin gene has only three exons and is about 1.5 kilobases (i.e. 1.5 thousand base pairs or 1.5 kb) long, while the huge dystrophin gene, in which mutation can give rise to Duchenne muscular dystrophy, has 60 exons and is 2000 kb long.

DNA sequences that perform essential functions often differ very little between individuals, and even between species, because mutations in such sequences are usually harmful and are eliminated by natural selection. These are called "conserved" sequences. About 60% of human proteins (and genes) are conserved, while about 40% of proteins are polymorphic, i.e. they may differ to a small extent between individuals. The latter are responsible for most of the normal range of human variation; they may also be related to differences in predisposition to late-onset disorders. Intergene regions, by contrast, vary widely between individuals because changes in non-coding sequences often have little or no effect. Individual differences in repeating sequences are very common, and form the basis of "genetic fingerprinting"; variations in mitochondrial DNA have been used to trace the origin and dispersal of the human race. The inheritance of all types of individual variation can be traced in families, and such family histories are often very useful in genetic diagnosis.

Though unrelated individuals differ by millions of single bases and there are thousands of differences in the number of units in repeating sequences, the DNA from all human beings has a similar basic arrangement and organization. The concept of the "human genome" is based on this characteristic pattern of the DNA of the human species.

2.2 Genetic basis of diseases

2.2.1 *Chromosomal abnormalities*

Two full chromosome sets are required for balanced gene expression leading to normal embryonic development and functioning. However, errors of cell division leading to aneuploidy (one or more chromosomes present in too many or too few copies) are common during gamete formation. Aneuploidy usually causes failure of fertilization or of early embryonic development, or miscarriage. Only a few fetuses with abnormalities such as an additional chromosome 21 (Down syndrome), 18 (Edward syndrome) or 13 (Patau syndrome), or an additional or missing sex chromosome, survive to birth. The frequency of chromosomal aneuploidy, and hence of spontaneous abortion and of chromosomally abnormal infants, increases with maternal age.

Chromosomal rearrangements, in which two chromosomes exchange unequal portions of their DNA, can also occur during gamete formation, and are another important cause of genetic disease.

2.2.2 *Point mutations*

Its double-stranded structure makes the DNA molecule very stable, but single-base changes often occur spontaneously; these changes are termed point mutations. The natural mutation rate is increased by exposure to mutagens such as ultraviolet light, radiation or chemical carcinogens. Even the smallest change causes a mismatch between complementary strands and distorts the DNA helix. In most cases DNA is repaired by enzymes that recognize distortions, cut out the "wrong" base, and replace it with the correct one. Mutations are the rare changes that escape DNA repair, and, since this is most likely to occur during DNA replication, spontaneous mutations usually arise at cell division.

There is thought to be about one mutation per cell division, with most mutations occurring in somatic cells. Most have no effect or lead simply to cell death, but those involving growth-controlling genes sometimes lead to cancer.

Mutations in germ cells are also usually harmless, but some can cause genetic disease in the offspring or more distant descendants. The full range of possible types of mutation is very wide, ranging from single-base changes to the insertion or deletion of several bases. Changes in the number of repeat sequences adjacent to genes can also affect gene functioning. Mutations in a coding sequence can lead to production of an abnormal protein; thus sickle-cell haemoglobin is the result of a specific, single-base change in the β-globin gene. By contrast, a wide variety of different mutations in adjacent non-coding sequences involved in normal gene functioning can cause underproduction or absence of the relevant protein. For example, β-thalassaemia can be due to any one of more than 100 different mutations in and around the β-globin gene, and cystic fibrosis is caused by any of more than 400 different changes in and around the cystic fibrosis transmembrane conductance regulator gene.

Point mutations arise more often during the formation of sperm, which continues throughout life, than of ova, in which cell division is completed in the embryo. The frequency of many new mutations therefore rises with paternal age.

2.3 Genetic diagnosis

A hereditary component in disease can be detected in a variety of ways. There may be a family history of a particular condition, with or without a typical mendelian inheritance pattern (although conditions may also cluster in families for environmental reasons). The condition may be associated with the presence or absence of a particular protein and hence with an abnormality of the corresponding gene. The use of modern molecular methods may reveal an association between the particular disease and specific changes in DNA.

When a genetic disorder is diagnosed in one member of a family, the concern immediately arises that other family members may carry the same gene, develop the same disorder, and hand it on to their children. Relatives need clear information about such risks, which calls for correct diagnosis in the affected family member and reliable methods for detecting symptomless carriers.

Genetic diagnosis starts with inheritance pattern. Severe disorders with a characteristic clinical picture due to a mutation in a specific gene (e.g. Huntington disease, haemophilia, phenylketonuria (PKU)) follow fairly clear-cut inheritance patterns that directly reflect the transmission of the abnormal gene. These are the single-gene disorders with classical mendelian inheritance (Fig. 5). However, a simple inheritance pattern is the exception, since most clinical disease categories are broad and complex, and some mutations are harmful only in certain circumstances. Clinical categories of disease that have a genetic component but that are not always due to mutation in the same gene have a multifactorial inheritance pattern, i.e. may show some familial aggregation but no typical mendelian pattern.

2.3.1 Single-gene disorders

Single-gene disorders are important causes of fatal or chronically disabling disease, especially in childhood, and have led to the development of the modern biochemical and DNA methods now being used for investigating the genetic component in more common and complex disease categories.

The main mendelian inheritance patterns are shown in Fig. 5. Since all genes are liable to mutate from time to time, the number of single-gene disorders is very large: more than 6000 are now known (1). Individually,

Figure 5
Classical mendelian patterns of inheritance

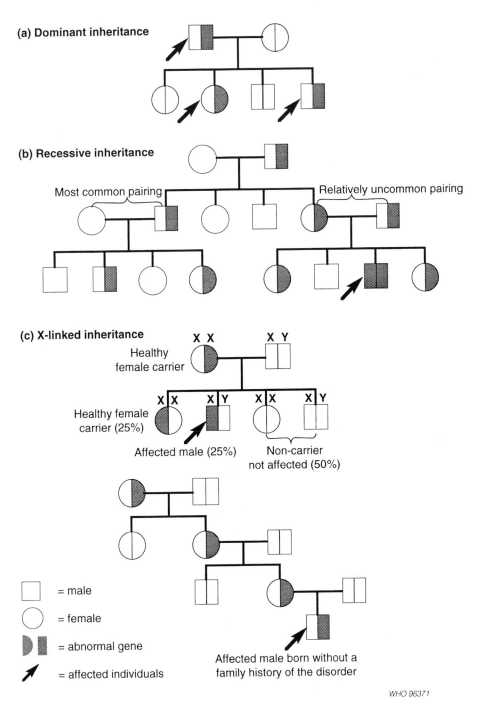

(a) Dominant inheritance

(b) Recessive inheritance

Most common pairing   Relatively uncommon pairing

(c) X-linked inheritance   X X   X Y

Healthy
female carrier

X X   X Y   X X   X Y

Healthy female
carrier (25%)

Affected male (25%)   Non-carrier
                           not affected (50%)

☐ = male

◯ = female

◗ ▮ = abnormal gene

↗ = affected individuals

Affected male born without a
family history of the disorder

WHO 96371

Note: Explanatory legends on p. 10.

9

Legends to figure 5 on page 9:

(a) *Dominant inheritance.* Everyone inheriting a gene for a dominant disorder is likely to be affected. Severe, early-onset dominant disorders (e.g. osteogenesis imperfecta or brittle bone disease) are usually caused by new mutations, arise without a previous family history, and are not passed on to descendants because they are fatal in early life. Parents of an affected child have a very low risk of the disorder recurring in subsequent pregnancies. Dominant conditions transmitted in families are usually of late onset, after reproductive age is reached (e.g. Huntington disease, adult polycystic disease of the kidney, family cancer syndromes, tuberculous sclerosis, neurofibromatosis). Carriers of dominant genes have a very high reproductive risk; each of their children has a 50% chance of inheriting the gene and suffering from the same disorder.

(b) *Recessive inheritance.* Recessively inherited disorders include haemoglobin disorders, cystic fibrosis, phenylketonuria and Werdnig-Hoffman disease. Carriers are healthy themselves but have a reproductive risk. When partners carry the same mutated gene, there is a 1 in 4 chance in each pregnancy that the child will suffer from the disorder. Most people carry one or two lethal recessive mutations, but these are usually transmitted through many generations without causing disease. Most children with a recessively inherited disease do not have a family history. About 50% of their first-degree relatives will be carriers, but only a tiny fraction of the carriers present in the population can be identified by testing family members. Therefore, when a condition is common and carrier screening is feasible and useful, it is appropriate to offer it at the population level.

(c) *X-linked inheritance.* Most mutations on the X chromosome are transmitted through unaffected carrier females (with two X chromosomes) and affect mainly, but not exclusively, males. Examples include haemophilia, Duchenne muscular dystrophy, fragile X mental retardation and glucose-6-phosphate dehydrogenase deficiency. In principle, about 60% of carriers of X-linked disorders might be detected by family studies, but a family history may be absent if the disorder has been transmitted in the female line for several generations or is the result of a new mutation. Female carriers are at high genetic risk; in each pregnancy there is a 25% risk of an affected son and a 25% risk of a carrier daughter.

most such disorders are rare, but collectively they are quite common. However, just a handful of the most frequent conditions may account for almost half of all single-gene disorders worldwide.

Specialist clinical and laboratory expertise is needed to diagnose single-gene disorders. Given a correct diagnosis, the known inheritance pattern of a particular disorder allows information on risk to be given to affected individuals and their relatives. When the gene involved is known, it may be possible to offer definitive carrier tests (biochemical or DNA) to determine which relatives are, and which are not, carriers of the mutated gene. Carriers may then be able to follow one of a number of courses of action to avoid handing the disorder on to their offspring (see section 6).

2.3.2 *Multifactorial disorders*

An increasing number of common disorders are recognized as having a genetic component, either because of evident familial clustering or because of an association with a specific form of a protein or specific DNA sequences.

Some common multifactorial disorders considered to be due to the interaction of several genetic and/or environmental factors are discussed in section 4. Among these disorders, some will be due to genetic causes alone, some to environmental causes alone and some to both. A baby with neonatal jaundice, for example, may have one or more of the following genetic or environmental problems: prematurity, infection, G6PD deficiency, rhesus incompatibility, congenital hypothyroidism or an inherited disorder of bilirubin metabolism; jaundice will be exacerbated by breast-feeding. The genetic component is beginning to be similarly understood in other multifactorial disorders, including congenital malformations, coronary heart disease, diabetes mellitus, asthma and cancer.

A small minority of cancers (family cancer syndromes) are clearly inherited; these include familial polyposis coli, familial non-polyposis colon cancer and some thyroid cancers. Familial cancers are usually due to inherited mutations in a single growth-controlling gene and show a dominant, late-onset inheritance pattern. The inherited single mutation does not cause disease in itself but, when a new, spontaneous mutation inactivates the remaining normal gene in a relevant tissue cell, cancer can arise. Better understanding of the mutations underlying familial cancers is also improving understanding of the commoner forms of cancer, and could lead to the recognition, and subsequent control, of environmental carcinogenic stimuli.

Most common cancers are due to sporadic mutations affecting growth-controlling genes. Some cancer-causing mutations would happen regardless of the individual's circumstances, and others may be related to environmental carcinogens or factors such as smoking and diet. There is now also known to be a major genetic component in cancer of the colon and the breast, although in these relatively common conditions it can be difficult to distinguish familial from non-familial cases.

In a disorder such as cancer or coronary heart disease, features that should arouse suspicion of an inherited predisposition include:

- early onset
- similarly affected parents and/or siblings
- when there is a difference in frequency between the sexes, occurrence in the less commonly affected sex (e.g. coronary heart disease in women).

The existence of a multifactorial disorder in an individual or a population does not necessarily imply the presence of abnormal genes. Many multifactorial disorders seem to be due to interactions between a genetic constitution within the normal range of human variation and the environment. For example, some HLA (histocompatibility leukocyte antigen) types that are highly protective against specific infections also predispose to autoimmune disorders (insulin-dependent diabetes mellitus (IDDM), ankylosing spondylitis, haemochromatosis). In a given environment, random combinations of such variants can result both in individuals with a particularly robust constitution and in others who suffer from specific disorders. A change of environment may reverse the situation. This may, for example, partly explain the high prevalence of non-insulin-dependent diabetes mellitus (NIDDM) in many populations that have changed rapidly from a traditional to a modern lifestyle, although *in utero* environmental factors may also be involved (p. 32). Thus there is a tendency for each family to recognize an individual health profile that shapes its members' expectations in terms of longevity and particular health problems. The Human Genome Project is making it possible to identify such genetic variants, and the appropriate use of this information presents a major new medical challenge.

2.4 Advances in molecular genetics

DNA technology depends on a number of basic tools that have been gradually developed over the past 20 years or so. A wide range of enzymes involved in DNA and RNA synthesis and repair have been identified and become available for laboratory use, nucleotide bases are available as laboratory reagents, and specific DNA sequences can be synthesized at will. DNA diagnostic methods have been greatly simplified over the past 10 years, and rapid progress continues to be made in this area.

DNA has many advantages for genetic diagnosis. It is easy to obtain, since every cell of an individual or fetus contains the full DNA complement of that individual. Genes can be studied whether they are actively producing their product or not. A definitive diagnosis can usually be made, and essentially similar laboratory approaches can be used for the diagnosis of all genetic conditions. One important limitation of DNA diagnosis, however, is that many different mutations may underlie the same clinical disorder, and it can be difficult to identify them all, particularly the rarer ones.

2.4.1 *DNA technology*

Major new techniques that are contributing to the advances in medical genetics include the following:

- The synthesis of DNA probes with specific sequences that will bind to and identify any complementary DNA sequences that may be present. This allows genetic diagnosis and permits further analysis of DNA by the examination of unknown sequences adjacent to the known ones.
- DNA sequencing methods for the rapid analysis of unknown DNA and the identification of mutations that give rise to disease.
- New diagnostic techniques, such as the use of restriction enzymes that cut DNA consistently only at specific sequences, and the polymerase chain reaction (PCR) for amplifying known DNA sequences. Such methods allow simple and rapid diagnosis using extremely small tissue samples. It is even becoming possible to analyse the DNA contained in a single cell.
- Techniques for synthesis of DNA that allow the production of known sequences of increasing length. Coding sequences produced in this

way can be used for the production of therapeutic agents such as insulin, erythropoietin and factor VIII. They may also be used in the creation of transgenic animals and in gene therapy.

- Positional cloning strategies using genetic markers, which are now defined along the entire human genome. These have greatly simplified the study of families. Even quite small kindreds can be examined using highly informative probes, and disease mutations can be rapidly assigned to their chromosomal position.
- *In vitro* methods for examining the protein product of gene sequences with unknown functions.
- New cytogenetic techniques such as fluorescence *in situ* hybridization (FISH), which permits direct visualization of the relationship of genes to one another in the nucleus of the living cell.
- Comparison between the DNA sequences of different genes and species. This helps elucidate the mechanisms of evolution.
- Insertion of coding DNA sequences into animal embryos to create transgenic animals, including animal models of human diseases. The availability of transgenic techniques and the use of experimental site-specific mutagenesis are particularly valuable for studying the roles of specific genes in multifactorial diseases, where combinations of different genotypes and environments can be examined.
- Insertion of missing DNA sequences into individuals with genetically determined disorders, or the excision of harmful sequences (gene therapy).

Some of these technologies (particularly gene amplification by PCR) are easy to use and inexpensive, and ideal for international studies.

Much of the new information about human genetic disorders obtained by such techniques has been both unexpected and of fundamental importance. For example, it is now clear that several inherited neurological diseases (e.g. fragile X mental retardation, Huntington disease, dominant cerebellar ataxia, spinal bulbar muscular atrophy and myotonic dystrophy) are caused by the amplification of short repeating sequences adjacent to genes essential for normal brain development and function. The best-studied example to date is the fragile X mental retardation gene (FMR-1), which was located in 1992, although its protein product is still unknown. The fragile X mutation is a large increase in the length of a normal CGG repeat sequence adjacent to the gene, which arises in two separate steps. Some individuals carry a "premutation", in which the number of CGG repeats is increased from the normal 10–50 to as many as 200 copies, but have no clinical problems. Occasionally, however, during female gamete formation, the sequence expands further to a "full mutation" with over 600 repeats; this inactivates the FMR-1 gene, locally disrupts the chromosome structure, and leads to mental retardation. DNA diagnosis and carrier testing are now possible, both prenatally and in mentally retarded children and adults.

It has also been found that the expression of some DNA sequences depends on whether they were transmitted through the male or female parent. For example, one particular sequence causes Prader–Willi syndrome if inherited from the mother but gives rise to Angelman syndrome if inherited from the father. This phenomenon is known as genetic imprinting. A category of disorders caused by inheritance of mitochondrial mutations from the mother has also been defined. There are likely to be many more unexpected findings, particularly in relation to how genes interact with each other and the environment in the development of the nervous system and the brain.

2.4.2 *The Human Genome Project*

The Human Genome Project is an attempt to systematize the research on mapping and isolating human genes that is already in progress in many countries, in order to create a single linear map of the human genome, with each coding gene defined and sequenced.

The primary aim of the Human Genome Project is to advance knowledge rather than to identify disease mutations. Its most important outcome will be to increase understanding of the way in which genes interact with each other and with the environment to generate normal structure and function. The findings will also cover the individual variation that incidentally contributes to susceptibility to common diseases. The definition of intergene and control regions will improve understanding of neurological and embryological development, with potential implications for the prevention of congenital abnormalities and mental retardation. Progress will be greatly facilitated by the use of genetically engineered animal models and new, highly sensitive, cytogenetic techniques.

The importance of the Human Genome Project for human health should be neither overestimated nor underestimated. DNA data obtained by mapping and sequencing will need to be correlated systematically with clinical and scientific data, which may be more difficult to obtain. Once relevant genes and their interactions with each other and the environment have been defined, scientific, clinical, epidemiological and psychological research will be required to determine gene function and to identify possibilities for prevention or treatment of particular disorders. International collaboration is essential to ensure that clinically relevant information can be applied worldwide, and to permit international and interregional comparisons, quality control, technological simplifications and free exchange of reagents and clinical data.

The burden of congenital and genetic disorders is frequently greatest in developing countries (see section 3) where the emerging health problems often have a genetic component. It is important to encourage genetic studies in populations with specific problems (such as the thalassaemias in Asia and the Eastern Mediterranean, sickle-cell disease in sub-Saharan Africa, and non-insulin-dependent diabetes in Polynesia), to ensure that technology and resources are generally available and to maintain international collaboration. It is an important function of the Human Genome Organization (HUGO) to ensure that data from the Project are available to all, in an integrated and usable form.

Agencies with a role in coordinating human genome data include UNESCO, the Genome Data Base, HUGO, the National Institutes of Health/Department of Energy (USA), the Medical Research Council (UK), Genethon (France) and the European Union.

2.4.3 *The Human Genome Diversity Project*

As part of the work of HUGO, the Human Genome Diversity Project is aimed at increasing understanding of human evolution. The major objective is to define the genetic relationships between human populations and interpret them in terms of natural selection, genetic drift, migration, etc. For example, the frequency and distribution of rare single-gene disorders are related to the history of human migration. Differences in distribution between populations may often be accounted for by "founder effects". When a population expands from a relatively few founding members, some contribute more, and some less, to the genetic make-up of subsequent generations. If one prolific founder carries a genetic abnormality, this can lead to a localized cluster of affected individuals. Studies of isolated and aboriginal populations can be particularly informative. The Finnish population, for example, which was initially relatively small and isolated, has grown to several millions in recent centuries, without substantial immigration or admixture. Approximately 24 recessive diseases that are rare elsewhere are unusually frequent in Finland, and some that are common elsewhere in Europe (e.g. PKU) are absent. This suggests that the particular recessive genes for hereditary disorders that were present by chance in the "founder" population have multiplied proportionately. In addition, limited mobility, leading to the selection of marriage partners within areas of high gene frequency, has resulted in a relatively high birth rate of infants with these recessive diseases. With increasing population mixing, however, the frequency of affected infants is falling.

DNA methods are particularly helpful in investigating mutant gene distribution. For example, PKU is caused by mutations in the phenyl-alanine hydroxylase (PAH) gene. Five common mutations are found in the European population, and differences in their relative frequencies throughout Europe suggest a single major founding event in a specific ethnic group.

The Human Genome Diversity Project is not concerned primarily with health, but certain aspects of human genetic diversity related to health and disease are relevant to the Project. For instance, differences between populations in the incidence of common disorders such as hypertension, atherosclerosis, diabetes and some forms of cancer, and in the proportion of fit elderly people, suggest that the study of "genes for health" could be considered as part of the HUGO strategy.

2.4.4 *Relevance of new genetic knowledge for treatment: gene therapy*

Gene therapy is the introduction of a gene sequence into a cell with the aim of modifying the cell's behaviour in a clinically relevant fashion. It may be used in several ways, e.g. to correct a genetic mutation (as for cystic fibrosis), to kill a cell (as for cancer) or to modify susceptibility (as for coronary artery disease). The gene may be introduced using a virus (usually a retrovirus or adenovirus) or by means of lipid or receptor targeting. All these approaches have certain disadvantages; viral vectors, for example, are efficient in promoting uptake but may cause pathogenicity, and only a relatively short length of DNA can be introduced, while lipid and receptor systems are relatively inefficient in promoting the uptake and expression of DNA. However, there seems little doubt that new gene delivery systems will be developed, combining the advantages of existing systems but without their disadvantages.

There is now almost universal agreement that gene delivery to somatic cells to treat disease is ethical, and that gene therapy should take its place alongside other forms of medical treatment. It is useful to think of gene therapy as a way of using genes pharmacologically, and thus as being comparable to other forms of drug treatment. Because it will usually involve introducing a copy of a normal gene into cells, it may ultimately be safer and more amenable to biological control than many existing pharmacological approaches. Like all new treatments, gene therapy should be properly tested for safety and efficacy before general application in clinical practice. It does not appear to require any special regulations, but does need to be brought clearly into the normal system for the licensing of medicines and approval by the ethics committees that govern the introduction of new clinical products. The ethical aspects need to be coordinated internationally to ensure that the same general level of regulation is applied everwhere; otherwise, there is a risk that trials will be carried out only in places with less rigorous standards.

The Scientific Group was aware that, at the time of its meeting, clinical trials were proceeding in two areas, although all were at a very early stage; the trials were concerned mainly with monitoring toxicity, dosage and efficacy rather than with definitive treatment. Of these trials, the first concerned several hundred cancer patients in gene therapy research programmes designed to investigate the use of genes to enhance the toxicity of chemotherapeutic agents or increase tumour suppressor gene activity. The second involved a small number of patients with single-gene disorders that seem particularly suitable for study, including immune deficiency due to adenosine deaminase deficiency, cystic fibrosis and familial hypercholesterolaemia. Trials are foreseen for many other inherited disorders, including thalassaemia, sickle-cell disease and haemophilia. There is considerable interest in the possibility of somatic gene therapy for common disorders including diabetes mellitus, coronary heart disease and autoimmune disorders.

Many small biotechnology companies are starting up in the field of gene therapy, and established multinational pharmaceutical companies are also interested. Much of the technology is subject to patent protection, and many genes have also been patented, which may raise problems of equitable access to therapy in the future. It may become necessary to draw up an internationally agreed list of "non-patentable genes" to protect the right of access to gene therapy. It is important to ensure that access is not restricted only to those who have the ability to pay, particularly as the underlying technology is essentially simple, cheap and applicable worldwide. Several international organizations have recommended facultative patenting, to guarantee a return for a useful invention or therapeutic application, rather than restrictive patenting of gene sequences for which no use has yet been established.

It is important to remember that fundamental understanding may assist diagnosis but may not necessarily lead to treatment. For example, the exact DNA sequence of the human immunodeficiency virus has been known for years, but this knowledge, although valuable in diagnosis and epidemiology, has not so far been helpful for treatment. Haemoglobin genes were the first to be identified and sequenced; the information has already proved useful for prenatal diagnosis but not yet for treatment. Because some genes (e.g. in the brain) are very inaccessible and some have irreversible developmental effects, it must be expected that gene therapy will evolve slowly and will not necessarily be applicable to all conditions.

Although most public attention has been accorded to the possibility of gene therapy, the new genetic knowledge also permits the development of conventional forms of therapy, including protein and small molecule delivery (as for treatment of diabetes mellitus or emphysema), and environmental modification to lessen the risk of disease (e.g. hyper-cholesterolaemia). Such "low-technology" approaches could be inexpensive and applicable in all countries. Thus the new techniques of human molecular genetics are becoming an increasingly important component of the general health care strategy of many countries.

2.5 Conclusions

Rapid advances in gene mapping make it almost certain that the application of new genetic knowledge will dramatically increase the requirement for genetic approaches to the control of a wide spectrum of diseases, and provide possibilities for prevention and treatment of those diseases by changes in lifestyle and diet, periodic check-ups or gene therapy. Since the field of medical genetics now covers common diseases as well as the classical inherited disorders, all countries need to invest in genetic diagnosis and counselling.

3. Epidemiology of genetic disorders and service needs

In every community, priorities for medical approaches to the genetic component of disease will depend on local frequencies of relevant disorders, the health burden that they represent, the possibilities for prevention and treatment, the resources available and the health infrastructure. Disorders with a genetic component can be of any degree of severity and have their onset at any stage in life. However, those presenting at birth are particularly burdensome, as they may cause early death or lifelong disability.

3.1 Congenital abnormalities and genetic disorders

A congenital anomaly is defined as any structural, functional or biochemical abnormality present at birth, regardless of whether or not it is detected at that time. This definition covers the overlapping categories of genetic disorders and congenital abnormalities.[1] The best available figures on the incidence of congenital anomalies obtained in studies in developed countries are presented in Tables 1–3. Accurate prevalence data are difficult to collect because of the great diversity of disorders and because many that cause early death remain undiagnosed in the absence of specialist services. Moreover, not all such conditions are detectable at birth, and the proportion of the population known to be affected therefore increases with age.

Table 1 shows that, in a typical developed country, congenital and genetic disorders are the second most common cause of death in infancy and childhood (2). Table 2 shows the important contribution of these disorders to chronic childhood disability (2). In developed countries, the birth incidence of infants with congenital disorders, including those that are trivial or relatively easily corrected, is about 25–60 per 1000 (3); the more rigorously the data are collected, the closer the estimates come to the higher figure.

Approximate incidence figures are given in Table 3 for different categories of genetic disorder and congenital abnormality up to the age of 30 years in a typical developed country (4). If multifactorial conditions of late onset such as thyroid disease, diabetes mellitus, psychoses, hypertension, myocardial infarction, ulcers and familial cancers are added to these figures, it is estimated that 60–65% of the population will suffer from a genetically determined disorder during their lifetime (4, 5). This is not surprising: if major environmental causes of death (such as infection, accident, starvation and war) are avoided, people must die of their constitutional, often genetically determined, limitations. Genetic predisposition to disease is attracting increased medical attention as its

---

[1] Strictly speaking, the term congenital abnormality includes congenital malformations (genetic), disruptions (teratogenic) and deformations (caused mechanically *in utero*).

Table 1
Contribution of genetic and congenital disorders to infant and child mortality in a typical developed country[a]

Main causes of death at < 1 year[b]	%	Main causes of death from 1 to 4 years[c]	%
Perinatal factors	38	Accidents	31
Congenital and genetic disorders	25	Congenital and genetic disorders	23
Sudden infant death syndrome	22	Neoplasms	16
Infections	9	Infections	11
Other	6	Other	9

[a] Based on data for the United Kingdom for 1986 and 1987 (2).
[b] 9.6/1000.
[c] 0.9/1000.

Table 2
Importance of the genetic component in chronically disabling congenital disorders in a typical developed country[a]

Type of disorder	Incidence per 1000 births	Genetic component
Mental handicap:		
severe	3.5	Most
moderate/mild	25.0	Up to 30%
Cerebral palsy	2.5	Very small
Blindness	0.6	50%
Deafness (severe)	≈ 1.0	> 50%
Congenital anomalies	> 50	≈ 50%

[a] Source: reference 2.

importance in determining *premature* onset of common disorders is being recognized (p. 29).

It is reasonable to assume that the figures given in Tables 1–3 will apply, at least approximately, worldwide. In addition, however, the factors described below will increase the incidence of genetic disorders in many developing countries.

Demographic factors influence the incidence of *chromosomal disorders,* because of their relationship to advanced maternal age (Fig. 6). Where women continue having children up to the end of reproductive life, the birth incidence of children with chromosomal disorders may reach 6/1000, and of children with Down syndrome about 3/1000. When couples plan their families, the proportion of older parents usually falls very markedly, and there is evidence that this change alone has reduced the incidence of Down syndrome in European countries by 30–60% (6).

Table 3

Incidence of genetic disorders and congenital anomalies up to the age of 30 years in a typical developed country[a]

Category	Estimated births per 1000	Commonest diagnoses
Single-gene disorders		
dominant	7.0	Familial hypercholesterolaemia
		Adult polycystic disease of the kidney
		Huntington disease
		Neurofibromatosis
		Chondrodystrophy
X-linked	1.33	Muscular dystrophy
		Haemophilia and Christmas disease
		Colour vision disorders
		X-linked mental retardation
		Glutathione deficiency
recessive	1.66	Cystic fibrosis
		Phenylketonuria
		Amino-acid disorders
		Werdnig–Hoffman disease
		Thalassaemias
Chromosomal	3.49	
autosomes	1.69	> 70% Down syndrome
sex chromosomes	1.8	Mostly Klinefelter and Turner syndromes
Congenital abnormalities	52.80	
genetic component	26.60	Congenital heart disease
		Club foot
		Congenital dislocation of the hip
		Pyloric stenosis
		Cleft palate/lip
no genetic component	26.20	–
Other multifactorial	10.06	Strabismus
		Inguinal hernia
		Epilepsy
		Diabetes
		Mild mental retardation
Genetic, unknown type	1.20	–
Total genetic	51.34	
Total genetic + non-genetic congenital anomalies	77.54	

[a] Source: reference 4.

Haemoglobin disorders and *G6PD deficiency* are the commonest single-gene disorders in many, if not most, of the conurbations of northern Europe and America (6): over 4% of the global population carry a haemoglobin disorder, and more than 7% carry a gene for G6PD

Figure 6
Birth incidence of children with Down syndrome and other chromosomal disorders as a function of maternal age

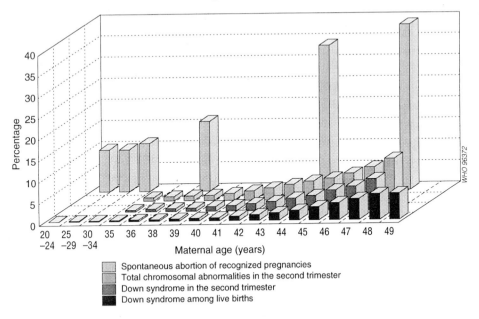

deficiency (*7, 8*). These high figures have been reached because carriers are protected against *Plasmodium falciparum* malaria: both types of genetic disorder are endemic in the tropics and subtropics, and migration has distributed them worldwide. The global distribution of these disorders has been mapped (Figs 7 and 8), and estimates of birth rates are available (*9*). Because of their high incidence and the burden of treatment, the haemoglobin disorders are often the first genetic condition to be recognized as a public health problem in developing countries. Comprehensive control programmes have been developed in many countries, and guidelines for their organization are available (*7, 9*).

Consanguineous marriage (marriage between cousins) is favoured by at least 20% of the world's population, and probably more, and it is estimated that, worldwide, at least 8.4% of children have related parents (*10*). The custom has existed throughout the Eastern Mediterranean region and in southern India, and among many tribal populations throughout the world, for thousands of years. Its distribution has been mapped (Fig. 9).

Customary consanguineous marriage is an important element in the social fabric of the communities in which it is practised, and can be supportive to women and the family. However, it also increases the birth incidence of children with recessively inherited disorders. For unrelated couples, the general risk of stillbirth, neonatal or childhood death, or serious congenital malformation is about 2.5%, and there is an additional

Figure 7
Global distribution of haemoglobin disorders, in terms of births of affected infants per 1000 births

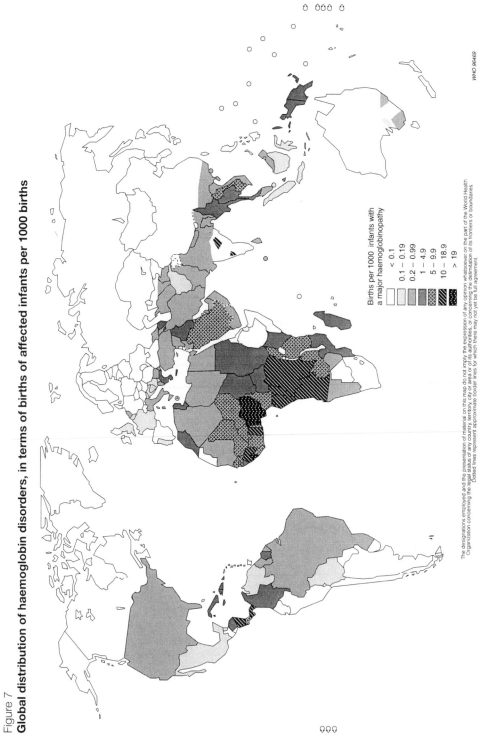

Births per 1000 infants with
a major haemoglobinopathy

< 0.1
0.1 – 0.19
0.2 – 0.99
1 – 4.9
5 – 9.9
10 – 18.9
> 19

The designations employed and the presentation of material on this map do not imply the expression of any opinion whatsoever on the part of the World Health
Organization concerning the legal status of any country, territory, city or area or of its authorities, or concerning the delimitation of its frontiers or boundaries.
Dotted lines represent approximate border lines for which there may not yet be full agreement.

WHO 96469

Figure 8

Global distribution of G6PD deficiency, in terms of the percentage of hemizygous males in the population, i.e. those carrying a deficient gene on their single X chromosome

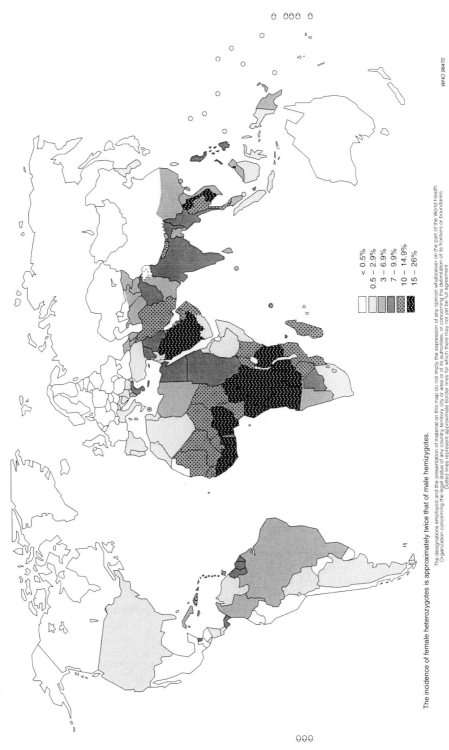

< 0.5%
0.5 – 2.9%
3 – 6.9%
7 – 9.9%
10 – 14.9%
15 – 26%

The incidence of female heterozygotes is approximately twice that of male hemizygotes.

The designations employed and the presentation of material on this map do not imply the expression of any opinion whatsoever on the part of the World Health
Organization concerning the legal status of any country, territory, city or area or of its authorities, or concerning the delimitation of its frontiers or boundaries.
Dotted lines represent approximate border lines for which there may not yet be full agreement.

WHO 96470

23

Figure 9
Global distribution of the custom of consanguineous marriage[a]

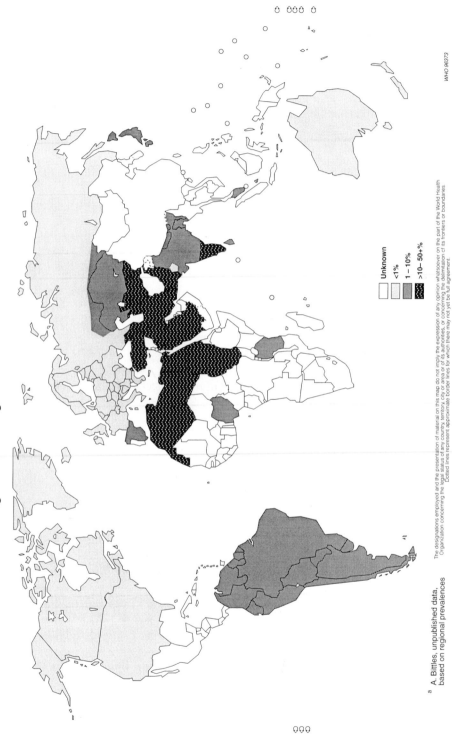

	Unknown
	<1%
	1 – 10%
	>10– 50+%

a A. Bittles, unpublished data,
  based on regional prevalences

The designations employed and the presentation of material on this map do not imply the expression of any opinion whatsoever on the part of the World Health
Organization concerning the legal status of any country, territory, city or area or of its authorities, or concerning the delimitation of its frontiers or boundaries.
Dotted lines represent approximate border lines for which there may not yet be full agreement.

WHO 96373

(almost 3%) risk of some degree of mental retardation. These risks are considered to be approximately double for couples who are first cousins. Where the infant mortality rate is high an effect of this order is barely noticeable, but when infant mortality falls (as it has done throughout the Eastern Mediterranean) congenital abnormalities and chronic disabling childhood disease may become more apparent. Appropriate genetic counselling in relation to customary consanguineous marriage is discussed in section 6.

Table 4 shows that these additional factors may increase the burden of childhood genetic and congenital disorders in many developing countries and among some ethnic minorities in more developed countries. Priorities for developing genetic services may therefore differ considerably between populations.

Susceptibility to common multifactorial disorders also appears to show important ethnic differences. In general, the frequency of coronary artery disease, hypertension and diabetes mellitus is increasing in developing countries as traditional practices are replaced with a lifestyle closer to that of developed countries. To some extent, these changes in disease frequency probably reflect differing genetic predispositions. However, there is also considerable evidence that an adverse environment before birth or in the early years of life can cause long-term physiological changes that predispose to coronary heart disease, hypertension or lung disease in later life. Such factors, combined with genetic predisposition, could be particularly important in populations that progress from relative malnutrition to dietary abundance within the space of one or two generations.

3.2 Management of congenital and genetic disorders

Table 5 summarizes the results of the treatment of congenital anomalies in typical developed countries. Overall, even under the best conditions, about 30% of affected children may be expected to die in infancy, about 40% may be successfully treated (largely by surgery) and about 30%, mostly with genetic diseases, will suffer from chronic severe disability. Many congenital abnormalities with potentially severe lifelong effects (e.g. squint, club foot, congenital dislocation of the hip, inguinal hernia, undescended testicles) can be corrected relatively simply, provided that basic paediatric services are available. Specialist paediatric surgeons can correct many more. Many abnormalities, however, particularly those of the heart and central nervous system, cannot be corrected and lead to lifelong disability and early death. It is possible to reduce the effect on mortality, disability and reproductive fitness in only 30% of single-gene disorders (11), though some of the commonest (haemoglobin disorders, cystic fibrosis and PKU) can be managed with considerable success. In summary, about 50% of congenital abnormalities, 10% of inherited diseases and 2% of chromosomal disorders can be successfully managed or corrected.

Table 4
Frequencies of congenital disorders: effect of additional factors in a number of countries[a]

Country	Maternal age (chromosomal disorders)[b]	Haemoglobin disorders[c]	G6PD deficiency[d]	Consanguineous marriage[e]	Additional disorders	Total disorders
Bahrain	3	8.46	5.10	8.25	24.81	101.1
Greece	–	1.75	2.58	–	4.33	80.6
Nigeria	3	19.20	6.00	+[f]	28.20	104.5
Pakistan	3	0.90	1.65	10.00	15.55	91.9
Thailand	–	4.80	3.15	–	7.95	84.3
United Kingdom	–	0.18	+[f]	0.05	0.23	76.5
USA	–	0.20	0.90	–	1.10	77.4

[a] The figures shown are per 1000 births.
[b] Estimated from maternal age distribution (*Demographic yearbook*. New York, United Nations, 1991).
[c] See reference 9.
[d] Estimated as 6% of male hemizygotes (8).
[e] Estimated as 25/1000 × proportion of first-cousin marriage (10).
[f] Frequency unknown.

Table 5
Estimated outcome for different types of congenital anomaly in typical developed countries[a]

Category of anomaly	Approx. no. of births[b]	Main therapeutic needs	Outcome		
			Early mortality (%)	Chronic problems (%)	Successful treatment (%)
Severe congenital malformation	30	Paediatric surgery	22	24	54
Chromosomal disorders	3.2	Social support	34	64	2
Inherited diseases	7	Medical management and social support	58	31	11
Total	40.2		29	28	43

[a] Estimates based on references *5* and *12*.
[b] Per 1000.

Management is often very burdensome for the patient, the family and society in general, and may have considerable implications for health service resources. As long as there is no effective treatment (as for Huntington disease, Duchenne muscular dystrophy and Werdnig-Hoffman disease), the proportion of patients in the population remains approximately constant. However, when management increases patient survival, the number of patients needing treatment increases cumulatively. For example, in the absence of prevention, the number of people in Europe with cystic fibrosis, PKU and haemoglobin disorders would increase more than fivefold over the next 50 years (*6*). In the Islamic Republic of Iran, more than 1000 children with β-thalassaemia major are born each year, and over 14 000 are now being treated at different centres. Each child requires at least 20 units of blood and about US$ 3000 worth of the iron-chelating drug desferrioxamine annually (*9*), amounting to an additional annual need for 40 000 units of blood and US$ 3 million for desferrioxamine. Such considerations highlight the importance of prevention and of research directed towards radical cure, including gene therapy.

Treatment and prevention are thus complementary aspects of services for genetic disorders. Families at risk need both types of service, as do communities: prevention programmes can "contain" the number of affected people and so permit communities to provide a standard of care that might not otherwise be possible. A systematic effort to combine prevention and treatment for a genetic disorder at the community level is described as a "control programme" for the disorder (*12*).

3.3 Prevention

Possible prevention approaches include: basic public health measures such as providing access to family planning, optimal maternal nutrition, prevention of infections, etc. (see section 5); genetic diagnosis and family counselling; early diagnosis and treatment when possible (e.g. for congenital malformations, PKU, congenital hypothyroidism, sickle-cell disease); and prenatal diagnosis. It has been estimated that use of all these approaches could prevent more than 75% of congenital abnormalities (*13*), but to combine such diverse preventive measures requires careful service planning and coordination.

3.4 Conclusions

To provide a basis for the treatment and prevention of genetic disease requires the following: basic demographic and epidemiological data to identify priorities; facilities for genetic diagnosis; care for the disabled and for children with chronic disease; preventive approaches; professional education designed to ensure that genetic approaches are incorporated into most branches of medicine; and audit, based on registers of congenital malformations, of patients with avoidable conditions and of prenatal diagnoses.

4. Role of genetic predisposition in common disorders

Research related to the Human Genome Project will eventually lead to the identification of every gene that contributes to susceptibility or resistance to disease. Common disorders such as coronary heart disease are influenced by several different genetic risk factors and, in the absence of increased environmental risk, people with a genetic predisposition may escape disease or develop it only at a relatively late age. It may therefore be valuable to identify such people so that they can adopt a healthy lifestyle and diet. It may also be wise to promote similar preventive measures for the whole population but, as these are unlikely to be adequate for people with a pronounced genetic predisposition, both a "high-risk" approach and preventive strategies for the whole population are indicated.

The following discussion of present knowledge of the genetic component in selected common conditions shows the large scale of the likely implications for medicine, the rapid rate of progress at the molecular level and the reasonable hopes for treatment and prevention aroused by recent developments. It also highlights the need for good prospective clinical, epidemiological and intervention studies, for improved provision of information to the public and for the integration of simple genetic approaches, including the taking of a genetic family history, into everyday medical practice.

4.1 Coronary heart disease

Although familial hypercholesterolaemia was already well known in the 1930s, until recently it was generally believed that environmental factors alone cause coronary heart disease. However, a careful family history will often uncover genetic susceptibility to coronary heart disease: the occurrence of premature coronary heart disease (e.g. myocardial infarction before the age of 55 years) in a relative, for example, confers a significant risk. Progress in mapping the human genome will greatly facilitate the detection of genetic predisposition to coronary heart disease and contribute to the understanding of atherosclerotic/thrombogenic processes at the molecular level.

About 25 years ago, evidence started to accumulate that risk factors such as serum cholesterol and blood pressure are genetically influenced, and that familial hyperlipidaemias confer an increased risk of coronary heart disease. Risk factors identified more recently include high levels of fibrinogen and possibly also of homocystine (both of which are genetically influenced), high levels of Lp(a) lipoprotein (not detectable by measuring cholesterol or other traditional lipoprotein parameters), and the apolipoprotein E4 (apoE4) polymorphism of apolipoprotein E. Non-apolipoprotein "candidate" genes (e.g. angiotensinogen-converting enzyme I) have also been identified.

The practical value of these developments depends on the extent to which they enhance the scope for treating and preventing coronary heart disease. A combination of risk detection and lifestyle counselling, with drug treatment when indicated, might in itself reduce the incidence of myocardial infarction to the low level of two or three generations ago. Gene therapy may become possible for some serious genetic causes, including homozygous familial hypercholesterolaemia, which is due to the absence from cell surfaces of low-density lipoprotein receptors. Other possible molecular approaches include "anti-sense treatment",[1] amplification of natural processes or the administration of substances that counteract disease development.

4.2 Cancer

Certain cancers, such as retinoblastoma and polyposis coli, are caused by major single genes, but most show no hereditary tendency. With such relatively common conditions, it can be difficult to distinguish between sporadic and familial cases, but it is now thought that a genetic pre-disposition may be involved in as many as 10–25% of cases of cancer of the colon or breast. At least one relatively common gene, probably on chromosome 17, is known to predispose to breast cancer. There is, however, a general lack of awareness of the importance of genetic factors

---

[1] Anti-sense treatment is the neutralization of harmful mRNA or DNA sequences by administering complementary sequences that selectively bind and inactivate them.

in cancer; a careful family history is rarely taken, and the existence of affected relatives is often missed.

Work on the human genome is identifying numerous genes that may affect susceptibility to tumour development. The genes for polyposis coli, familial non-polyposis colon cancer, retinoblastoma and neurofibromatosis have all been identified. Better understanding of these genes may lead to a general improvement in the diagnosis and treatment of cancer; for example, a DNA screening test for susceptibility to breast cancer could soon become available. However, the psychological as well as the clinical costs and benefits of such testing will have to be very carefully assessed.

The usefulness of detecting cancer susceptibility will depend on the effectiveness and acceptability of the preventive measures available. A primary objective is regular surveillance of the relatives of an index case so as to permit early detection of disease before irreparable local damage or metastasis has occurred. However, if a specific carrier test is not available, relatives may be faced with difficult decisions: many are naturally reluctant to consider potentially disfiguring surgery, such as prophylactic mastectomy or colectomy, on the basis of a 50% risk or less, but waiting for clinical evidence of risk may endanger their lives. One useful application of an understanding of cancer at the molecular level is likely to be the development of DNA methods for definitive carrier diagnosis. Research is now being focused on assembling cohorts of people with a family history of, for example, breast cancer, to permit long-term studies of genetic risk, the feasibility of identifying carriers, the value of surveillance (e.g. by regular mammography) and the psychological effects of these approaches.

When the results of current studies are known it may become possible to offer advice on the "chemoprevention" of cancers, tailored for families with different types of cancer risk. At the population level, people known to be at risk of contracting cancer of the lung should be advised not to smoke. Advice on healthy diet may help reduce the risk of gastric and colon cancers. There has been a very significant drop in the frequency of gastric cancer among populations of European origin over the past 30–40 years, which may be related to dietary changes, but it is difficult to draw confident conclusions at present, because the specific dietary changes involved are uncertain.

4.3 Asthma

Asthma and allergy have a strong familial tendency, and a specific gene that affects plasma levels of IgE may contribute to susceptibility. Knowledge of predisposition to asthma and allergies could have practical application in allowing people with specific susceptibility to abstain from exposure that could provoke disease or discomfort. Certainly a susceptible person would be well advised not to become a baker, for example, as it may be impossible to make a bakery sufficiently free of allergens to be a safe workplace. A concern often voiced about taking the results of genetic tests into account when choosing an occupation is that employers might be tempted to scale down their efforts to improve the working environment. However, in view of the benefits of avoiding or delaying the onset of disease, test options should be available to individuals, but employers (or prospective employers) should not be given access to test results.

4.4 Diabetes mellitus

Diabetes mellitus occurs in all populations. However, the incidence of insulin-dependent (IDDM) and non-insulin-dependent (NIDDM) diabetes mellitus varies considerably with age, country and ethnic group. Both types are associated with premature mortality and a high risk of vascular, renal, retinal and neuropathic complications.

Evidence for a genetic element in IDDM comes from studies that show a higher concordance in identical twins (25-30%) than in non-identical twins (5-10%). Genes on the short arm of chromosome 6, either within or close to the major histocompatiblility (HLA) region, are primarily responsible for genetic predisposition, which may operate through an autoimmune mechanism triggered by specific infections. A search for other relevant genes continues. As yet there is no indication for general population screening. However, if it were shown that diabetes linked to HLA polymorphisms could be prevented by immunizing susceptible people against the relevant infections, or if methods were developed to prevent the destruction of pancreatic islet tissue during such infections, population screening for genetic susceptibility could be indicated.

As the prevalence of IDDM is 3-6% among first-degree relatives of people with the disease, compared with 0.2-0.5% among the general (Caucasian) population, the former may be considered a high-risk group. A useful first step may be to identify carriers of a predisposing gene. People who will later develop diabetes can often be recognized by the presence of immunological markers and a decline in pancreatic β-cell function during the "prediabetic" stage of disease evolution. There is some evidence that "resting" the pancreas by giving short courses of insulin therapy may delay the onset of overt disease. At present, therefore, there is a reasonable rationale for careful, family-based, primary prevention studies designed to arrest the development of IDDM.

About 85% of cases of diabetes in developed countries are cases of NIDDM, which has a particularly strong familial tendency. The uncommon form found in adolescents and young adults (maturity-onset diabetes of the young) shows a dominant inheritance pattern. However, identification of susceptibility genes has been slow. Many patients with NIDDM exhibit insulin resistance and hyperinsulinaemia in association with dyslipoproteinaemia, central obesity, hyperuricaemia and high blood pressure. The prevalence and pattern of this cluster vary among different ethnic groups, and the extent to which it represents a single disease process is still uncertain. It has recently been linked to adverse environmental conditions before and after birth. As already mentioned, NIDDM is particularly prevalent – affecting up to 35% of adults – in some populations that have changed rapidly from a traditional to a modern lifestyle (American Indians, Pacific Islanders, Australian Aborigines and migrant Asian Indians).

Gestational diabetes mellitus is the name given to diabetes in women who first develop glucose intolerance during pregnancy. It occurs in about 3% of pregnancies in developed countries and, although there seems to be no excess of perinatal mortality or congenital malformations, the child of an affected mother is at increased risk of macrosomia. The mother herself is at increased risk of later developing NIDDM.

The aim of preventive strategies is to decrease insulin resistance and promote and sustain pancreatic β-cell function, e.g. by reducing obesity and promoting physical activity. Few published studies have so far shown an effect of preventive measures on the development of NIDDM, and such measures are probably most usefully applied to the following high-risk groups:

- individuals with a strong family history of NIDDM, especially of the early-onset type;
- populations in transition from traditional to more modern lifestyles, from rural to urban societies or from active to sedentary occupations;
- women with a history of gestational diabetes or of high-birth-weight infants;
- individuals with other elements of the "chronic metabolic syndrome", e.g. hypertension, dyslipoproteinaemia and obesity (particularly central obesity).

Diabetes of all types is an important candidate for future biological treatments, such as gene therapy or the transplantation of pancreatic tissue.

4.5 Mental disorders

Some mental disorders occur preferentially in people with an inherited predisposition. However, the relevant genes have so far proved extremely elusive and reported associations between genetic markers and, for example, schizophrenia have not been reproducible. It is possible that a large number of genes predispose to mental disease, so that consistent associations are hard to detect. Knowledge of increased risk of mental disorders might be of limited value at present, because there seem to be few possibilities for prevention. However, prevention can be studied only if people at risk are identified, and research, particularly at the molecular level, may yield unexpectedly useful results. In addition, some people could find the information useful in making reproductive choices.

4.6 Alzheimer disease

Alzheimer disease is a form of dementia associated with the presence of neurofibrillary tangles in neurons and senile plaques in the extracellular parenchyma of the brain. It shows a strong familial tendency and is known to be caused by at least four different genes. Knowledge of the genetics of Alzheimer disease is already casting light on pathological processes at the molecular level, and this may lead to ways of interfering with these processes. Prevalence of the disease, which is about 1.3% at age 69, rising to about 50% by age 95, has been increasing steadily in developed countries as average survival has increased. Familial cases are sometimes due to a mutation of the amyloid precursor protein on chromosome 21 but are more frequently related to genes on chromosome 14. Recently, a strong association has been found between the apoE4 polymorphism on chromosome 19 and late-onset Alzheimer disease. The apoE4 protein may participate in the disease process, and homozygotes are at very high risk of developing Alzheimer disease by the age of 80.

It is hoped that knowledge of the pathology of Alzheimer disease could be used to prevent or delay onset. For example, if apoE4 is involved, it may be possible to develop a drug to prevent the interaction of apoE4 and other components that gives rise to the characteristic brain lesions. Alternatively, if apoE3 protects against the development of Alzheimer disease, it might be possible to transfer the apoE3 gene to the somatic cells of people at risk.

4.7 Conclusions

Recent progress in molecular genetics has shown that inherited predisposition is important in a number of common diseases normally manifest in later life, such as atherosclerosis, coronary heart disease, hypertension, diabetes mellitus and some rheumatic, oncological and mental illnesses, which appear at an early age and develop into severe disabilities in predisposed people.

Enough is already known of the genetics of common diseases to introduce a family-oriented approach into basic as well as specialist medical practice. A major effort will be made in the foreseeable future to study the genetic factors in common diseases, develop appropriate therapies and determine how these approaches can best be applied in practice.

5 Approaches for prevention

This section is concerned with the application of approaches for prevention based on public health measures, genetic family history and genetic population screening.

5.1 Basic public health measures

Some important congenital and genetic disorders can be prevented by providing information for both the public and health workers and by making basic diagnostic facilities available. At present, these approaches tend to be integrated into routine antenatal care, but there is a growing appreciation of the need for preconception screening and counselling (see section 5.4.4).

Routine screening of women for *rhesus blood group* allows appropriate management of at-risk pregnancies; maternal immunization is prevented by giving Rh-negative women anti-D antibody after childbirth, miscarriage or termination of pregnancy.[1] Perinatal mortality and the chronic problems of rhesus haemolytic disease have fallen by over 95% in most developed countries as a result of appropriate management (6).

Congenital rubella is prevented by immunizing children and non-pregnant women and by testing pregnant women routinely for antibody; abortion[1] is usually offered to women infected in early pregnancy. The incidence of congenital rubella in western Europe declined from 3.5 to 0.41 per 100 000 births between 1980 and 1985 as a result of these measures (*14*).

Congenital toxoplasmosis can be prevented by advising pregnant women to eat only well-cooked meat and avoid contact with cat faeces. In some areas, vulnerable women are identified by antibody screening, followed by surveillance. Pregnant women and newborn infants with evidence of infection are treated with antibiotics to prevent damage to the eye or brain from primary or later reactivated infection.

The risk of *neural tube defects* can be reduced by giving the mother supplementary folic acid around the time of conception (*15*). In areas where neural tube defects are uncommon, dietary vitamin supplementation is recommended for women with a positive family history; in high-incidence areas, however, vitamin supplementation is now recommended for *all* women planning a pregnancy. In practice, only a small proportion of pregnant women are informed in time to increase their vitamin intake to the necessary extent.

Growing evidence that maternal health and nutrition affect predisposition to common disease later in life underlines the importance of preventing maternal anaemia and malnutrition. Pregnant women with *insulin-*

---

[1] See note on p. 2.

dependent diabetes have an increased (on average, 6%) risk of bearing a severely malformed child, but this risk can be greatly reduced by meticulous control of blood sugar, which should be started before pregnancy begins. A similar risk is associated with certain antiepileptic drugs. Mothers with either risk are candidates for expert scanning for fetal anomalies during the second trimester.

In populations where *G6PD deficiency* is common, the incidence of kernicterus and the need for exchange-transfusion can be greatly reduced by simple and inexpensive measures, such as screening of neonates, exposure of babies to light and educating the population not to feed broad beans (which will provoke a clinical reaction in G6PD deficiency) to children.

Stillborn infants and infants that die in the neonatal period should be examined by a paediatric pathologist to establish the presence or absence of a genetic problem. The parents can then be counselled on the risk of recurrence.

Public health approaches for the prevention of some common disorders with a genetic component are also being developed. Current understanding of the importance of environmental factors in the etiology of such disorders suggests that society as a whole should adopt a healthier diet and lifestyle. Truthful and realistic public information campaigns should be strongly supported. At the political level, measures to make a healthy diet and lifestyle economically rewarding may be considered, such as introducing standards for healthy food and imposing taxes on unhealthy foods or pastimes. The fall in mortality from coronary heart disease in many developed countries over the past few decades may reflect the control of several risk factors as the result of improved public information.

5.2 Detection of genetic risk

In order to prevent genetic disorders, it is necessary to identify people at risk of developing a disorder themselves and/or of passing a disorder on to their children. The two main approaches to identifying risk depend broadly on whether a condition is inherited or occurs sporadically.

Sporadic disorders include most congenital malformations and chromosomal disorders; the vast majority of affected children are born to parents with no known risk factor, and the risk of recurrence is low. There is usually a moderately increased risk for people with an affected relative (1-6% in most multifactorial disorders, 1-2% for chromosome disorders), and some other relatively high-risk groups can be identified (e.g. older women and women with IDDM). Since everyone is at risk for sporadic disorders, population screening (see section 5.4) using simple and reliable mass methods is the most effective preventive approach. Table 6 shows the objectives of different types of genetic population-screening programmes.

Table 6
Objectives of different types of genetic population-screening programmes

Type of programme	Primary objective	Secondary objectives
Preconception screening	Reducing risks to the health of the fetus	Informed reproductive choice
Antenatal screening	Identification of at-risk couples and affected fetuses in time for possible abortion[a]	Diagnosis of affected fetus, and prenatal or neonatal treatment
Neonatal screening	Case-detection for early treatment	Data on disease incidence
General population screening	Identification of high-risk factors	Prevention, early diagnosis and treatment of common diseases

[a] See note on p. 2.

Inherited disorders affect a limited number of families and are usually transmitted by healthy carriers who have a high risk of passing the disorder on to their children. Genetic counselling can be offered following the diagnosis of either genetic disease or the carrier state in a family member. In recessively inherited diseases, such as the haemoglobin disorders, most affected infants are born without a family history; however, the birth of an affected child identifies a family in which many carriers may be found. Most experience of genetic counselling to date is with single-gene disorders, but a "family-oriented" approach is now also appropriate for many other common disorders.

Genetic counselling can have the greatest impact when individuals or couples at genetic risk are identified prospectively, i.e. before they have developed symptoms themselves or produced their first affected child. Prospective counselling is technically possible only when carriers can be accurately identified. When suitable carrier tests are available, population screening can be used to identify people at risk in the absence of a family history. Most such screening is currently done in the context of reproductive risk, but screening for personal risk is likely to become at least equally important. To some extent, the established genetic population-screening services listed in Table 7 may serve as models for the development of future genetic screening programmes.

The effectiveness of a family-based approach is compared with that of population screening in Table 8. The increased power of population screening (when it is feasible and properly conducted) greatly enhances its significance at the public health level, especially as such services can be relatively inexpensive and highly cost-effective (p. 49).

Once a preventive service has been introduced, people who subsequently develop an avoidable disorder, or have an affected child whose birth

Table 7
Established genetic population-screening services

Type of service	Conditions	Preventive or screening action
Primary prevention	Rhesus haemolytic disease	Postpartum use of anti-D globulin
	Congenital rubella	Immunization of girls
	Congenital malformations	Addition of folic acid to the maternal diet (may prevent neural tube defects)
		Control of maternal diabetes
		Avoidance of mutagens and teratogens such as alcohol, certain drugs and possibly tobacco
Antenatal screening	Congenital malformations	Ultrasound fetal anomaly scan, maternal serum alpha-fetoprotein estimation
	Chromosomal abnormalities	Noting maternal age and maternal serum factor levels
	Inherited disease	Checking family history
		Carrier screening for haemoglobinopathies, Tay–Sachs disease
Neonatal screening	Congenital malformations	Examination of the newborn for early treatment (e.g. of congenital dislocation of the hip)
	Phenylketonuria, congenital hypothyroidism, sickle-cell disease	Biochemical tests for early treatment

Table 8
Proportion of affected pregnancies detectable by a family-based approach and by population screening

Type of disorder	Screening method	Estimated % detectable	
		Family-based approach	Population screening
Major congenital malformations	Fetal anomaly ultrasound scan	≈ 10	> 70
Down syndrome	Maternal age Maternal age plus maternal serum screening	30 –	– ≈ 60
Dominant and X-linked disorders	Family studies and carrier testing	30–60	Higher than in family-based approach
Recessive disorders	Carrier testing	< 10	Up to 100

could have been avoided, face much greater difficulties in accepting and coping with illness. Once it has been decided to establish such a service, there is an ethical obligation to make it widely and rapidly available.

Although the family-based approach and population screening differ in basic concepts, strategy, financial implications and associated ethical issues, the two are complementary rather than mutually exclusive. Taking a genetic family history is a screening method for identifying families with a genetic disorder who may benefit from referral to an expert. When a new test is developed that might be useful for population screening purposes, it is usually applied first in the families of affected people, and the decision on whether or not to extend screening to the whole population is based on the results obtained.

5.3 Genetic family studies

A characteristic feature of medical genetics is that a genetic diagnosis has implications for whole families as well as for individuals. While a correct diagnosis benefits individual patients, who can be given guidance on the management, natural history and prognosis of the particular condition and put in touch with appropriate support groups, it is also of value to other family members, who can be offered genetic counselling.

Counselling is necessary to counter false beliefs about hereditary disease (e.g. that the woman is responsible) and to relieve anxiety. In Nigeria, for example, it has been shown that genetic counselling alone greatly improves the quality of life of families and patients with sickle-cell disorders, as measured by improved school attendance, decreased maternal anxiety and increased parental acceptance of the affected child (O. Akinyanju, personal communication).

Relatives often also benefit from counselling about their own risk and the options available both for themselves and for their descendants. Relatives at risk, of whom a high proportion may be carriers, can be identified from the family history and should be offered genetic counselling. Many people, both with and without an affected relative, are concerned about possible genetic risk and prefer to be informed about such risk if the knowledge can increase their control over their own health and that of their family. Relatives may wish for definitive carrier testing if suitable tests are available and if positive results can lead to useful avoiding action such as a modification of lifestyle to reduce the risk of a common disorder, regular surveillance where there is genetic susceptibility to cancer or prenatal diagnosis in the case of genetic reproductive risk. To ensure that relatives are offered help at the appropriate time, medical geneticists usually maintain genetic registers and adopt an outreach approach for contacting people who may be at risk.

Unfortunately, outside the context of specialist genetic clinics, the importance of genetic counselling and family studies is often forgotten amid the pressures of patient care. A study in a Dutch haemophilia clinic showed that only about half of the female relatives who might be carriers had been informed of their risk or offered testing (*16*); in many other circumstances the figure would be even lower.

Although "family-oriented preventive medicine" has long been practised by many good family physicians, the importance of genetic as well as environmental factors in many common disorders calls for a more systematic approach in general medical practice. This is currently under study in several centres devoted to the prevention of cardiovascular disease or cancer. Having a first-degree relative with early-onset coronary heart disease is a risk factor in its own right, and should ideally be sufficient reason for any person who so desires, together with close relatives, to become clients in a system of family-oriented preventive medicine. Dietary habits, lifestyle, body fat and blood pressure are carefully recorded. Blood tests may include the measurement of blood lipids or apolipoproteins, possibly including apoE, Lp(a) lipoprotein, fibrinogen, and possibly homocystine (p. 29); DNA markers are included as associations with disease risk become established. The risk of cardiovascular disease is then evaluated from the total information collected, and preventive advice is tailored to the needs of the individual and other family members.

The nuclear family is an important executive instrument in family-oriented preventive medicine since disease prevention becomes a joint project to which all the family members contribute. Most of the families involved have already had serious disease experiences, and many members are already anxious; appropriate information coupled with the physician/geneticist's plan for preventive action often eases anxiety and creates optimism and positive attitudes.

It is important to increase both professional and public awareness so that more families at risk are identified and referred. Some programmes work with young people in educational institutions, identifying increased risk of cardiovascular disease by collecting information on possible clustering in families. An extensive programme operating in Utah combines the collection of family information with the teaching of biomedical sciences; the students, in collaboration with their parents, other students and teachers, draw up and interpret pedigrees.

Greater emphasis on genetic counselling is needed in medical education and practice. The taking of a genetic family history should be included both in the training of doctors and nurses and in refresher courses for those already in practice.

5.4 Genetic population screening

A genetic population-screening programme is a systematic effort to identify and counsel as many people at genetic risk as possible. A simple "primary screening test" is usually offered to the whole population to identify those groups at increased risk who are then offered further tests until a definitive diagnosis is reached. Classically, in population screening, everyone is offered testing when they pass through a convenient "screening turnstile" where medical tests are routine, e.g. when a pregnancy is reported or during the neonatal period. Genetic population screening for the detection of reproductive genetic risk or the early detection of treatable genetic disorders in newborn infants is now an integral part of maternal and child health services. The various factors that have proved to be important in such genetic screening programmes, and will become even more important once screening for genetic predisposition to common disorders is available, are discussed below.

A screening programme is a public health policy. It needs systematic planning and the support of the public health authorities. The classical requirements (17) are:

- a common and potentially serious condition
- a clear diagnosis in each case
- sound knowledge of the natural history of the condition (so that the outcome with and without intervention can be correctly predicted)
- an effective and acceptable method of treatment or prevention
- affordable tests.

Genetic population screening affects very large numbers of people and, if inappropriate, can do more harm than good. It requires the same high standards of diagnosis, quality control and counselling as specialist genetic services. Safety and efficacy, false-positive and false-negative rates, and costs and benefits must be carefully assessed. Moreover, screening tests are usually developed at expert centres under optimal conditions which may not be achievable when tests are used more widely. Many practical problems must be solved, such as the education of all the participants, ensuring the regular collection, transport and storage of uncontaminated samples, efficient laboratory organization and quality control, and recording and communicating of results. Since the organizational requirements vary with the local health and social infrastructure, screening programmes should first be introduced as research projects that aim to solve practical problems in the area concerned and to meet accepted standards of quality.

5.4.1 *Experience with genetic screening programmes*

Simple and reliable carrier tests have long been available for haemoglobin disorders (9) and Tay–Sachs disease (18), and population screening programmes, including public education, counselling and prenatal diagnosis, have greatly reduced the birth incidence of these disorders. A flow-chart for screening for carriers of a recessive gene, as in haemoglobin disorders and other recessively inherited conditions, is shown in Fig. 10. Existing programmes have demonstrated the following important points:

Figure 10

Flow-chart for genetic screening and prenatal diagnosis for carriers of a recessive gene, indicating the non-financial benefits and costs of each step in the sequence

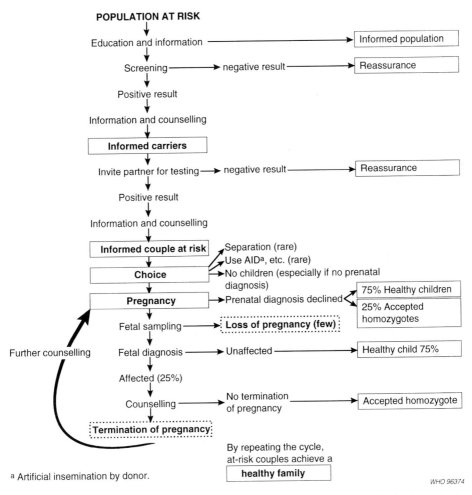

a Artificial insemination by donor.

WHO 96374

The main problem for couples found to be at risk is the unexpected or unwanted birth of a seriously affected child. The benefits of a screening programme are an informed community, informed carriers, informed choice for couples at risk, the birth of accepted affected infants, and the replacement of affected with healthy fetuses. The principal (non-financial) cost is the termination of a wanted, but affected, pregnancy. Similar charts could be drawn up for other screening programmes, but the starting point might be different, e.g. screening for the risk of Down syndrome in the fetus can begin only after pregnancy is established.

- It is possible to carry out a genetic screening programme efficiently, in an appropriate and socially sensitive manner.
- When adequate information and counselling are provided, identifying carriers of recessively inherited disorders does not cause serious psychological problems; most couples at risk prefer to have the information so that they can make careful reproductive choices.

- A successful programme depends on the involvement of the whole community; public information and preparation for screening are therefore essential.
- Large numbers of health workers in primary care and maternal and child health services require basic training in genetics and the principles of genetic counselling. Lack of such training is currently the main factor limiting the equitable delivery of these services.

5.4.2 *Screening of neonates*

Neonates should be routinely examined for congenital abnormalities, particularly dislocation of the hip, which can be simply corrected at this stage. The examination should be performed by an experienced paediatrician: inexpert handling can *cause* dislocation of the hip or necrosis of the femoral head. Ultrasound or sound transmission screening may prove safer and more reliable than clinical examination (*19*). Ultrasound screening during pregnancy can identify fetuses in need of paediatric surgery; delivery can then be arranged at a centre where specialist help will be immediately available.

Biochemical screening of newborn infants was first used for PKU in 1966 after it was shown that a low-phenylalanine diet started very early in life prevents severe mental retardation. Heel-prick blood samples are usually taken by midwives 5–10 days after birth. Several drops of blood are collected on filter paper (the Guthrie card), which is sent to a central screening laboratory. Once this system is established, screening for other conditions becomes relatively simple and cheap. Table 9 shows the disorders for which neonatal biochemical screening is (or can be) routine, and the false-positive rates of each test.

Screening of newborn infants for congenital hypothyroidism is carried out in most developed countries (*20*). It is also recommended for sickle-cell disease, which can be detected cheaply and reliably by haemoglobin electrophoresis (e.g. using Guthrie blood spots); early mortality can be reduced, and parents can be given genetic counselling (*21*). However, for every one affected child, haemoglobin electrophoresis also identifies around 40 carriers who need to be followed up because their parents may be at risk and in need of genetic counselling. Primary health care workers must be recruited to provide counselling regarding such common genetic traits.

Neonatal screening for cystic fibrosis is based on the measurement of immunoreactive trypsin in Guthrie blood spots. A positive result is now immediately followed by DNA studies for definitive diagnosis and to help to distinguish false-positives (*22*).

In general, the conditions listed in Table 10 fulfil the classical requirements for screening. As DNA technology improves the precision of genetic diagnosis, possibilities for neonatal diagnosis will certainly increase. For example, it is now possible to use a stored Guthrie card

Table 9
Neonatal biochemical screening tests

Disorder	Birth incidence	Neonatal assay/test	Positives (per 1000)	Detection rate (%)	False-positive rate (%)	Remarks
Phenylketonuria	1/10 000	Phenylalanine	0.3	98	60	Established value. Permits largely successful treatment
Congenital hypothyroidism	1/3 000	Thyroid-stimulating hormone	6.0	98	96	Established value. Permits successful treatment
Sickle-cell disease	0–1/100[a]	Haemoglobin electrophoresis	Varies with population	100	< 2	Established value. Avoids many infant deaths
Cystic fibrosis	1/2 000	Immunoreactive trypsin	–	–	–	Value uncertain. May improve prognosis. Permits genetic counselling
Duchenne muscular dystrophy	1/6 000[b]	Creatine phosphokinase	1.8	50–90?	96	Value mainly for genetic counselling
Congenital adrenal hyperplasia	1/10 000	17-hydroxy-progesterone	0.2–2	98?	95	Value in males clear. Little value in females with normal external genitalia
Congenital dislocation of the hip	1/400	Ortolani and Barlow manoeuvres	20	Varies with examiner	90	Requires expertise and repeated examination.

[a] In certain ethnic groups.
[b] 1/3000 boys.

Table 10
Routine antenatal screening tests[a]

Scan for fetal viability, number, gestational age

Blood tests, including:
  haemoglobin
  ABO and rhesus blood groups
  rubella antibodies
  hepatitis B virus
  human immunodeficiency virus

Carrier screening for:
  haemoglobin disorders
  Tay-Sachs disease
  cystic fibrosis

Maternal serum alpha-fetoprotein (AFP) or triple screen for risk of neural tube defects or Down syndrome
Routine fetal anomaly scan

[a] Includes all routine tests carried out at advanced centres. *Some* of these tests are provided for most pregnant women in most circumstances.

(which provides a small DNA store) to identify the genetic defect in a dead child, so that appropriate diagnostic procedures can be made available to the parents. As the possibilities increase, it will be necessary to consider how severe a condition must be to justify neonatal screening, whether the information that can be given will be sufficiently clear and whether the avoiding action that can be taken will be effective. For example, Duchenne muscular dystrophy usually becomes clinically apparent only in the second year of life, so some at-risk couples have a second affected child before the first has been diagnosed. The disorder can be detected simply and reliably in the newborn, but early diagnosis does not affect outcome. However, it has been calculated that, if all affected infants were identified early, family studies and genetic counselling could reduce the number of new cases by 15–20% (*23*). Research is in progress at several centres on the psychological implications and effects of neonatal screening for Duchenne muscular dystrophy.

Neonatal genetic screening requires a careful approach to counselling to avoid certain pitfalls, such as the accidental revelation of non-paternity. Moreover, it is essential to create a system that will ensure a genetic diagnosis remaining attached to an individual's medical records for life.

5.4.3 *Antenatal screening and prenatal diagnosis*

Screening pregnant women is an efficient approach to identifying reproductive risk, and is the only possible way to detect fetal chromosome disorders or malformations, which arise sporadically at or after conception. Table 10 lists the screening tests concerned with risk of genetic and congenital disorders that are now widely considered a routine part of antenatal care.

Risk of fetal chromosome disorders is the commonest reason for antenatal genetic screening. Amniocentesis for fetal karyotyping was initially offered to older pregnant women, i.e. maternal age was the initial "screen" that identified the group at increased risk who might then be offered definitive diagnosis. In developed countries, however, the proportion of older mothers is falling and therefore fewer fetuses with Down syndrome are detected in this traditional way. Hence there is great interest in developing better initial screening tests that can be offered to women of all ages. It has been found that the level of several measurable factors in maternal blood is altered when the fetus has Down syndrome. A "triple screen", in which assay of maternal serum alpha-fetoprotein (AFP), unconjugated estriol and human chorionic gonadotropin (HCG) is combined with maternal age and ultrasound examination, has been shown to identify a group of about 5% of pregnant women who carry about 60% of affected fetuses (24) and who can then be offered amniocentesis. Such testing is becoming widespread in more developed countries. Its disadvantage is that maternal serum screening can be done only at around 16 weeks of pregnancy and therefore leads to late prenatal diagnosis and late abortion[1] in the case of a positive result.

The best national data currently available on public attitudes to, and uptake of, antenatal genetic screening are contained in the report of the Canadian Royal Commission on New Reproductive Technologies (25). National surveys showed that a large majority of women favour the availability of services for prenatal diagnosis and termination[1] of pregnancy in the case of severe fetal abnormality. There was a wide range of individual attitudes towards termination but most women felt that this must be a personal decision and would use the diagnostic service themselves if they found that they were at risk.

According to the report, 6% of all pregnant Canadian women in 1990 (over 22 000) were identified as at increased risk of genetic disease in the fetus and were referred to genetic services for counselling and the offer of prenatal diagnosis. Advanced maternal age was by far the commonest reason for referral. Uptake of testing was 89% (10% of women either chose not to have a test or miscarried before testing). Of the 19 795 women tested, 95% received reassuring results. A fetal disorder was detected in about 990 cases, and 80% of the mothers concerned decided to terminate pregnancy. Decisions were strongly influenced by the severity of the chromosomal disorder diagnosed, as shown in Table 11.

The report also identified important inequities in the delivery of the genetic service. Marked interregional differences in the proportion of pregnant women referred were shown to be due to local variations in

---

[1] See note on p. 2.

Table 11
Mothers' decisions following prenatal diagnosis of fetal abnormality[a]

Type of disorder	Women terminating pregnancy[b] (%)
Trisomies 13, 18 and 21 (Down syndrome)	83
Neural tube defects	76
Turner syndrome (XO)	70
Klinefelter syndrome (XXY), XYY and XXX syndromes, balanced translocations, mosaics	30

[a] Source: reference 25.
[b] See note on p. 2.

Table 12
Limitations of antenatal screening

- The option of whether to undertake a pregnancy at all is no longer open
- Choice is unnecessarily urgent, difficult and painful
- Some women come too late for prenatal diagnosis to be possible
- Most women at risk are identified too late for first-trimester prenatal diagnosis
- Some carrier tests are more difficult to interpret during pregnancy
- There is no time to correct clinical or laboratory errors
- Hurried decisions may be regretted later
- Rapid staff turnover and lack of staff with specific responsibility for screening make a consistent policy difficult to achieve

doctors' perceptions of the importance of offering prenatal diagnosis, rather than to differences in women's attitudes.

Antenatal screening can have other important limitations (Table 12). If a diagnosis can be made by means of DNA, biochemical or cytogenetic tests, prenatal diagnosis can often be done by chorionic villus sampling (CVS) (p. 61) at about 9-10 weeks of gestation. The results are usually available early enough to allow the option of abortion[1] to be exercised before 12 weeks' gestation. Early prenatal diagnosis is far more acceptable to women than later testing (p. 59); when screening is confined to the antenatal period, most women at risk are identified too late for first-trimester diagnosis. In many countries, most women at risk for haemoglobin disorders, for example, are currently identified only in the second trimester of pregnancy. In these circumstances, only about 40% of women at risk for sickle-cell disorders request prenatal diagnosis, compared with about 80% of those informed of their risk during (or

[1] See note on p. 2.

before) the first trimester. Clearly, screening before conception, or at the earliest recognition of pregnancy, is desirable for carriers of inherited disorders, since they have a lifelong risk that is detectable at any time, may affect every pregnancy and has implications for other family members. Screening for inherited reproductive risk should therefore become part of primary health care, and maternal and child health services need to be strengthened in this important area.

5.4.4 *Preconception screening and counselling*

Women need information on the following topics *before* pregnancy:

- The significance of a family history of childhood death or disability, or premature onset of common disorders.
- The risk of miscarriage and fetal chromosomal abnormality, which increases with maternal age, and the availability of early prenatal diagnosis.
- The importance of balanced maternal nutrition for the immediate and long-term health of the baby.
- The effect of folic acid or multivitamin supplementation at or before the time of conception in reducing the risk of fetal neural tube defects and probably of other congenital anomalies.
- The importance of immunity to rubella.
- Possible indications for testing for specific genetic risks (e.g. rhesus blood group, haemoglobin disorders, Tay–Sachs disease, cystic fibrosis).
- The effects of smoking, alcohol consumption and medications for specific disorders in increasing the risk of miscarriage, congenital abnormality and fetal growth retardation.
- The importance of avoiding certain maternal infections that can harm the fetus (e.g. toxoplasmosis and listeriosis).

Preconception screening and counselling require: the establishment of a suitable infrastructure; improved medical and community education on genetic matters; freely available educational materials for women and health workers; basic training in genetic counselling for health workers; and the strengthening of laboratory diagnostic services.

The appropriate infrastructure will vary from community to community. Special preconception clinics tend to attract mainly educated, motivated individuals of middle socioeconomic class. In Hungary, however, pre-conception counselling has been provided through an "optimal family planning programme" developed over many years (26), and the service, run by nurses, is attended by more than 30% of young couples. It provides a framework for counselling and an ideal setting for prospective randomized studies, e.g. of the effectiveness of multivitamin supplements in preventing neural tube defects and other congenital abnormalities. It has also been found that a visit to the service provides a psychologically appropriate opportunity for other forms of health screening such as measurement of blood pressure and counselling about lifestyle. This type of service could provide a basis for screening for risk factors for common diseases in the future.

Where a family planning service exists, this may also be suitable for preconception counselling; many women seeking advice on family planning or birth-spacing are contemplating a future pregnancy. An apparently ideal infrastructure for preconception counselling already exists where family doctors provide family planning services.

5.4.5 *Screening for risk of common disorders*

Much more limited experience is available of the screening of adults for genetic predisposition to disorders that may affect their own health. The best example to date is screening for blood lipid levels, in particular total serum cholesterol, with a view to reducing the risk of coronary heart disease. Numerous lipid-screening programmes exist, some offering blood-lipid screening to all men of a certain birth cohort in a given region, and others aiming to screen specific groups independent of age or sex, such as employees in a given industry or people in certain professions or military or educational institutions.

The combination of family history, personal history and a small number of laboratory analyses already makes it possible to identify a substantial proportion of people at increased risk of contracting coronary heart disease. As additional genetic risk factors are identified, the potential for population screening is increasing rapidly. Susceptibility tests similar to those for coronary heart disease and dyslipidaemias may soon become available for several other disorders, including certain cancers.

Where the detection of susceptibility to certain diseases can lead to implementation of preventive measures, a rational attitude towards screening programmes should be encouraged. However, genetic predispositions are complex and, as with other tests, genetic screening can uncover unwelcome information. It is likely that polymorphisms related to common diseases have multiple effects, and caution is needed in initiating large-scale population screening.

The development of many other screening programmes for genetic predisposition is foreseen. As regards how and where this is to be done, much can be learned from screening programmes for non-genetic health risks. A dedicated screening programme may be appropriate when special technology is required (e.g. mammography), but the majority of screening (e.g. for cancer of the cervix, and routine recording of body mass index and blood pressure) takes place in the context of primary health care. Genetic screening may become an appropriate part of such health-promotion activities, especially in health systems where the primary care physician is a family doctor.

Information and testing are different aspects of disease prevention. Correct information carries negligible risks, is relatively inexpensive and should be provided at as many stages in life as possible, starting in school. Carrier testing, by contrast, can have serious implications and requires informed consent. There is no single ideal approach for genetic screening; a variety of different strategies are needed simultaneously.

5.5 Costs and benefits of genetic services

Although the incidence of many genetic disorders is low, they are among the most serious of medical conditions because many are fatal or cause chronic disability. Treatment, when effective, is therefore exceptionally beneficial in terms of years added to life or improved quality of life.

Even when no effective treatment is available, diagnosis and genetic counselling offer important benefits. Parents of affected children make huge efforts to obtain treatment, whether through public or private systems of health care. Correct diagnosis prevents a constant round of false hopes and useless treatments, increases acceptance of the situation, guides support for affected people and conserves family resources. Carrier detection and counselling offer people options for prevention, including the possibility of a "disease-free" family through prenatal diagnosis and abortion.[1]

Genetic diagnosis and counselling should be integrated into the growing range of available medical services, but will bring about an increased need for specialist genetic services to accept referrals. The cost–benefit ratio of providing such services, whenever it has been formally evaluated, has been shown to be extremely favourable in terms of health "bought" for funds expended (6). Since the broad benefits of genetic services are still not widely understood, such analyses have usually been presented primarily to health decision-makers to justify funding for programmes such as the provision of screening and prenatal diagnosis, and have – understandably – used money as the sole unit of measurement. Other costs and benefits have generally been ignored because they are so much more difficult to measure, with the result that an analysis might, for example, compare the cost of prevention by screening and prenatal diagnosis with the cost of treating a particular disease.

Cost-oriented analyses consistently show that prevention is cheaper than treatment but this approach is likely to cause considerable misunderstanding. Placing the main emphasis on the fact that caring for disabled individuals is costlier than preventing their birth is distressing to patients and their families, and conveys a message to the public that medical practitioners and health planners are lacking in compassion. It implies that the primary aim of the health system is saving money, rather than caring for patients, whereas this is not the real reason for physicians and health policy-makers supporting prevention programmes. Such programmes are supported because they enable people to lead better and more fulfilling lives, they reduce suffering, and they allow choice in one of the most important areas of life – that of having a healthy family. Their

---

[1] See note on p. 2.

principal benefit may therefore be described as the restoration of "reproductive confidence" to couples at risk. Such non-financial costs and benefits to both individuals and families, and to the larger society, must be the key elements in the objective evaluation and planning of genetic programmes.

As an example, Fig. 10 (p. 41) shows some of the non-financial costs and benefits of screening and prenatal diagnosis for a common recessively inherited disorder. Both treatment and prevention are included, since they are complementary, and every step has its associated costs and benefits. The benefits of a screening programme are an informed community, informed carriers and informed choice for couples at risk. The main non-financial cost is the termination of wanted, but affected, pregnancies.[1] Since the monetary cost of managing severe chronic disease is so great, the savings achieved by such programmes are bound to weigh heavily with health service planners, but should not be viewed as the primary objective.

5.6 Conclusions

There are now extensive – and generally cost-effective – possibilities for preventing congenital and genetic disorders, plus growing potential for the prevention of some common conditions with a genetic component. Many different approaches are involved, and, while only countries with a highly developed health infrastructure are able to apply *all* of them, some preventive actions are simple and cheap and thus suitable for inclusion in almost all health programmes. Government involvement is necessary if the implementation of such public health programmes is to be both effective and equitable.

6. Genetic counselling

6.1 Basic principles

Individuals and couples found to be at increased genetic risk need specialist services, but their access to such services depends on health workers – particularly those involved in primary health care – being sensitive to genetic risk. The basic principles of genetic counselling, the feasibility of incorporating counselling into primary health care, and the probable future requirements for counselling in connection with common diseases are discussed in this section.

Although counselling has a role in many areas of medicine, it is particularly important in the field of genetics because of the predictive nature of much genetic information, the psychological impact of knowledge of genetic risk for the individual, the implications for other

---

[1] See note on p. 2.

family members and the difficult decisions that people at risk often have to make. Genetic counselling is a skill that is best acquired by specific training. In addition to accurate genetic knowledge, it requires time and the ability to communicate. The main components are:

- A correct diagnosis.
- The estimation of genetic risk; this often requires a pedigree and may call for investigations involving other family members.
- The provision of information on existence of risk and on any options for avoiding it; options will depend on:
  - the nature of the disorder involved, the prognosis and the availability of treatment or palliative care;
  - the chances that other family members may be at risk and, in particular, of passing the risk on to children;
  - the possibility of avoiding risks to the individual's own health;
  - possibilities of avoiding transmission of the risk to children (techniques, problems, risk of error or complications).
- Accessibility for long-term contact; people at genetic risk may need counselling and support at several times in their lives.

Everyone who suspects a personal genetic risk or a risk of having offspring with a serious disease or malformation should have access to genetic counselling. Counselling will replace vague or incorrect ideas with correct information on risk, on particular disorders and on the availability of management and prenatal diagnosis. Relief of anxiety is a very important aspect of genetic counselling. For example, any couple who have had a child who died at an early age, had a child with a congenital disorder or know of such cases in the family are going to be worried that they could have a similarly affected child. Quite often, however, the disorder that worries them is non-genetic in character or has a negligible risk of recurrence; information to this effect can restore the couple's reproductive confidence.

In addition, genetic counselling can help people to deal with important risks that they may not have known about before. Positive results in carrier tests, particularly for dominant and X-linked disorders, can be disturbing, can lead to moral and psychological problems and can sometimes arouse anger and disbelief. Table 13 shows that the personal and reproductive implications for carriers of single-gene disorders differ with the mode of inheritance. It has been demonstrated that, given adequate information and counselling, diagnosing the carriers of recessively inherited disorders is not associated with serious psychological problems because there is no personal risk to carriers, their reproductive risk is relatively low and depends on the carrier status of their partner, and prenatal diagnosis is available.

By contrast, an individual is likely to find the knowledge of being a carrier for a dominantly inherited disorder very disturbing; the usefulness of that knowledge depends on the availability of effective ways for

Table 13

Mode of inheritance and personal and reproductive implications for carriers of single-gene disorders

Personal and reproductive implications	Mode of inheritance		
	Dominant	X-linked	Recessive
Psychological effects	+ +	+	Very small
Threat to personal health	+	0/±	0
Risk of having affected children	+	+	Potential only: depends on partner
Chance of an affected child if "at-risk" couple	50%	≥25%	25%
At-risk people can be identified by family history	Most	Many	Very few

preventing the development of the condition or for treating it. Familial hypercholesterolaemia, which confers a high risk of premature coronary heart disease, is a good example. Gene carriers can be identified on the basis of family history or by serum cholesterol screening. All available evidence indicates that the prognosis can be improved by changes in diet and lifestyle, together with the appropriate use of cholesterol-lowering drugs. However, such regimes call for intensive surveillance; in practice, they tend to have limited value because of non-compliance. Thus, even in the best circumstances, knowledge of carrier status is likely to be associated with uncertainties and anxieties. In addition, known carriers may find that they have restricted access to medical and life insurance, an important potential complication of screening for personal genetic risk. Carriers are also concerned about reproductive risks, and may need to discuss the advisability of having their own children if many family members have contracted myocardial infarction or died early, for example in their thirties.

Another classical, but less typical, example of a dominantly inherited disorder is Huntington disease, which can as yet be neither treated nor postponed. The tracing of the Huntington disease gene to chromosome 4 in 1983 made provisional carrier diagnosis possible. The exact mutation (an expansion of an adjacent variable (CAG) repeat sequence from the normal range of 11–34 copies to 42–66 copies) was identified in 1993, so that carrier testing can now be definitive. However, carrier (i.e. presymptomatic) diagnosis gives rise to serious psychological problems because of the absence of effective treatment. In practice, uptake of carrier testing is low, although the majority of family members say that they approve of it (27). Such testing is often requested to assist in planning reproduction or other aspects of life.

The identification of a woman as a carrier of a serious X-linked disorder (such as fragile X syndrome which causes severe mental retardation) also has important psychological as well as practical implications. Such a woman has a reproductive risk in every pregnancy, regardless of the genetic make-up of her partner, and is likely to feel solely responsible for any resulting problems for her children. Recent developments in DNA technology have generated an urgent need for more research in this area. It is now possible to screen mentally retarded individuals for fragile X syndrome so that genetic counselling may be offered to their relatives. It is also feasible, in principle, to identify every woman at risk of having an affected child but, before screening for the whole population can be contemplated, much more information is needed on the psychological impact on carriers, especially where mental retardation is concerned.

The difficult choices that can follow a genetic diagnosis are not limited to a few rare conditions; they arise quite commonly as a result of screening in modern pregnancy care, and involve most obstetricians, midwives and family doctors. A couple told after screening that they are at risk of bearing an abnormal child, or a pregnant woman who finds that she is carrying an abnormal fetus will have to choose one of the options shown in Table 14. All the choices have moral implications, and people need time and help to make the decisions that they feel are morally right. They must live with the consequences of their decisions for the rest of their lives and comprehensive and sensitive counselling will be essential.

There is little evidence of people taking genetic risk into account in choosing partners and none of an increased divorce rate among couples who discover a genetic risk after marriage. Numerous studies do show, however, that most couples wish to know of any risk of having children with a serious congenital disorder. Solutions such as adoption and artificial insemination by donor have not proved popular among couples confirmed as being at risk. When prenatal diagnosis is available, many take advantage of it; where it is not, most couples at high genetic risk would use it if it were (28). Prenatal diagnosis is thus an extremely important option for women and couples at genetic risk.

Because of the complexity of the situation and the fact that people faced by the same problem may make very different decisions, it is generally agreed that genetic counselling should be "non-directive". This does not mean, however, simply giving people the facts and leaving them to make up their own minds; rather, it implies that they should be actively helped to reach the decision that is right for them, in their personal circumstances and according to their own moral code, not that of the health worker.

In practice, therefore, genetic counsellors recognize the following three key principles (29), which provide useful guidance on most of the ethical questions associated with genetic diagnosis and screening:

Table 14

Options open to carriers of an inherited disease

Time at which risk is discovered	Possible action	Frequency
Before choosing partner (uncommon)	Remain single	Uncommon
	Avoid selecting another carrier as a partner[a]	Very uncommon
	Select a partner in the usual way	Most common
Before pregnancy (more common)	Remain childless	Common only for severe disease when prenatal diagnosis is impossible
	"Take a chance"	Common for less severe diseases
	Use prenatal diagnosis	Very common
	Use artificial insemination by donor or other form of assisted reproduction	Very common
	Separate and find another partner[a]	Very uncommon indeed
After birth of an affected child (most common)[b]	Accept infant and treatment	Usual
	Accept infant, but reject treatment	Occasional
	Reject infant	Occasional

[a] Relates only to recessively inherited disorders.
[b] The options that apply before first pregnancy also apply to pregnancies following the birth of an affected child.

1. The autonomy of the individual or couple is paramount.
2. The individual or couple has the right to complete information.
3. The highest standard of confidentiality must be maintained.

Genetic counselling takes time, and most clinical geneticists work with a number of trained associates (usually nurses, sociologists or biological scientists), who often bring additional skills to the consultation.

6.2 Genetic counselling in primary health care

Even in countries where clinical genetics is a recognized speciality and geneticists are assisted by counsellors, the large amount of basic genetic counselling now required cannot possibly be provided by specialist centres alone (6). The need to develop an appropriate structure for increasing the availability of genetic counselling in primary health care is now appreciated. Clinical geneticists have developed the necessary genetic knowledge, counselling skills and ethical, non-directive, family-centred approaches, which must now be integrated appropriately into many other branches of medicine. In North America there are now recognized, but non-medical, genetic counsellors with training equivalent to a master's degree. In other countries, there is a move to integrate genetic counselling into existing health services, including those for antenatal, family planning and primary care. This latter approach seems particularly appropriate when primary care is provided by family practitioners – usually the only clinicians apart from medical geneticists with a commitment to the family as a unit. However, integration of genetic counselling into primary health care requires regular in-service training and the support of experts; this may be most appropriately provided by specialist genetic counsellors, such as those already associated with most genetic services. Efficient and accurate genetic counselling in primary health care requires the development of a range of appropriate information materials for health workers, including leaflets, etc., that they can hand out to patients, plus audio- and videotapes, which may be even more useful than printed matter in such a complex area.

It is often said that genetic counselling takes too long to be possible in the context of primary health care. For example, carriers of common recessive conditions (e.g. haemoglobin disorders, Tay–Sachs disease, cystic fibrosis) need clear information about the following:

- the high incidence of the trait, and the fact that carriers are healthy and will not develop the disease;
- the pattern of inheritance (although it is not necessary to mention genes and statistics; most people are satisfied with a simpler explanation);
- the main features of the disease;
- the possible advantages of the carrier state, such as protection from malaria (see p. 21);
- the fact that relatives have a high risk of being carriers and might benefit from testing;
- the fact that knowledge of carrier status rarely influences people's choice of partner but may affect their reproductive behaviour;
- the existence of support groups, from which further help is available.

It is important to ensure that those concerned really understand that they are "healthy carriers" and do not, and never will have, the disease. Certainly this often takes longer than the 5–10 minutes of a routine consultation, especially as each person should be given time to reflect on what they have been told, and should be specifically asked whether they have any further questions. It is therefore desirable to identify particular primary care workers, such as midwives or nurses, for training in basic genetic counselling techniques. They should be able to set aside enough time to help people to absorb information and to make informed decisions when necessary, e.g. on whether to recommend testing to other family members.

Time will be saved if appropriate leaflets and other information materials are available *before* face-to-face discussions take place; encounters will be more fruitful if people have had time to decide what questions they would like to ask. Many excellent information materials can be obtained from support groups. Public information programmes and appropriate education in schools will also save time in genetic counselling: the better the community is informed the less the need for extensive face-to-face counselling. Thus, community education is not just essential, it is also cost-effective.

6.3 Ethical issues

Ethical aspects of genetic screening and counselling have recently been the subject of intense public interest and a number of authoritative reports have been produced. Section 9 of this report is devoted to ethics. However, a few ethical issues that arise quite commonly in genetic counselling practice call for separate discussion here.

6.3.1 *Customary consanguineous marriage*

There has been considerable uncertainty about how to provide genetic counselling in communities where consanguineous marriage is favoured. Should marriage to a relative be discouraged on genetic grounds, or is it possible to reduce genetic problems for families through a more sensitive and selective approach? Clearly, where consanguineous marriage is an integral part of the fabric of society, criticism must be avoided and people should be helped to preserve the advantages of customary marriage practices.

In most communities where the practice is common, consanguineous marriage can be supportive to women and hence to the family. In most such communities, families are "patrilineal"; that is, a woman leaves her own extended family at marriage to enter that of her husband. Cousin marriage can reduce the difficulties of this transition, because parents remain in contact with their daughter when she marries, and she is more likely to live nearby. In addition, equal numbers of sons and daughters are needed within the extended family; a daughter is therefore not perceived as a burden, and financial security is increased by the multiplicity of blood ties. In societies that practise segregation of the sexes, young couples can best get to know each other before marriage if they are related, and the expenses and exchange of property associated with marriage may be reduced.

In view of the foregoing, campaigns at the population level to discourage cousin marriage on genetic grounds seem inappropriate. In the first place, the vast majority of consanguineous couples will have perfectly healthy children; preventing such marriages may well do harm rather than good. Secondly, such an approach is contrary to the basic non-directive principles of genetic counselling. Thirdly, as in medicine in general, there are no "blanket" solutions; a selective approach designed to identify families at increased genetic risk and to provide them with appropriate genetic counselling is recommended.

It also seems, at least in theory, that genetic counselling might be particularly effective in communities where consanguineous marriage is common: when an affected person is diagnosed, family studies will allow other at-risk individuals or couples to be identified within the extended family and counselled before they themselves develop disease or have affected children. In this situation, therefore, it is even more important to train primary care workers to identify families with affected members and to refer them for expert genetic counselling.

6.3.2 *Who should decide?*

The basic principles of genetic counselling indicate that both the decision to undergo screening, and any consequent decisions, e.g. regarding prenatal diagnosis or termination of pregnancy,[1] should be made by *informed* individuals and couples. In an area where so many ethical uncertainties exist, the people who are themselves at risk may be considered the best judges of what should be done. It is they who often have first-hand experience of the condition in question and who, after considering the issues, must actually make the decisions that they will have to live with for the rest of their lives. The experience of genetic counselling shows that most people make highly responsible decisions, determined primarily by their personal perceptions of right and wrong.

The question of whether prenatal diagnosis (assuming that it becomes technically possible) should be permitted for risk of, for example, mental disease or diabetes often causes considerable concern. However, the above considerations show that such decisions should be made by the couples themselves, the health worker's main responsibility being to provide accurate, clear and comprehensive information. The way that the community as a whole actually uses genetic services can be observed by recording and reporting the choices that people make in practice, and these observations may be a better guide than speculation in determining the services that it is ethical to provide.

6.3.3 *Is it ethical to limit women's access to prenatal diagnosis?*

Prenatal diagnosis is an important option for women and couples at increased risk of having children with a serious genetic disorder; it should be available to as many such people as possible in countries where abortion on genetic grounds is legal. According to the ethical principles of genetic counselling, the choice for or against prenatal diagnosis should be made by the well-informed woman. However, a divergence of views between health workers and the people that they are counselling is not uncommon.

---

[1] See note on p. 2.

For example, a professional who is opposed to abortion may be unwilling to discuss prenatal diagnosis; it is generally agreed that the woman or couple must then be referred to someone who will offer access to this service. It is also common for obstetricians to make prenatal diagnosis available only to women who have already decided to terminate pregnancy[1] if a fetal abnormality is found, in view of the risk to the fetus. However, the ethical principles of genetic counselling dictate that prenatal tests should be available to *all* informed women who request them, even to those who are completely opposed to abortion; testing may provide reassurance, permit an informed choice to care for a disabled child or allow a mother to reconsider abortion.[1] In developed countries, in fact, most legal cases in this area have been initiated because a woman who was at detectable risk was *not* informed and offered testing and subsequently had an affected child.

At a more general level, it is sometimes feared that the increasing ability to predict genetic characteristics will lead to prenatal diagnosis and abortion[1] for minor, even frivolous, reasons. However, this greatly underestimates the seriousness with which people view the termination of a wanted pregnancy. There is no evidence of generalized abuse or overuse of prenatal diagnosis and selective abortion.[1] In the case of thalassaemia, informed choice has resulted in a marked reduction in the number of affected births. The same is not true, however, for all inherited diseases. Thus not all couples at risk for having children with sickle-cell disease choose prenatal diagnosis and, where the fetus has one of the less severe chromosomal disorders, the parents often choose to continue the pregnancy. When congenital malformations are detected by ultrasound scanning in early pregnancy, parents usually request abortion[1] only if the future for the fetus appears extremely grave.

6.4 Conclusions

An appropriate structure is needed for genetic counselling in primary health care, in which advantage is taken of the expertise of medical geneticists. At the same time, the recognized ethical principles of genetic counselling must be respected. Increased emphasis on genetic counselling is needed in medical training and practice. The taking of genetic family histories should be included in the training of doctors and nurses and in refresher courses for those already in practice.

---

[1] See note on p. 2.

7. Obstetric aspects of prenatal diagnosis

Prenatal diagnosis is now an integral component of obstetric care and genetic services in many countries. As a result of developments in ultrasound and DNA technology, more than 600 abnormalities could be diagnosed prenatally by 1992 (*30*).

A large proportion of women who know they are at increased risk of having a seriously disabled child request prenatal diagnosis, regardless of religious belief (*31*). When this service is not available, couples at high genetic risk often take steps to avoid pregnancy altogether, but will resume normal reproductive behaviour when testing becomes possible. Nevertheless, large variations in the utilization of prenatal diagnosis services have been observed. These depend to some extent on individual differences in the perception of the burden imposed by a genetic disorder, willingness to accept the risk, and legal, moral, emotional or religious objections to the termination of pregnancy. However, studies of prenatal diagnosis in Canada (*25*), and of its use for the haemoglobin disorders (*32*) show that the most important limiting factors are inadequate information for couples at risk, failure of the obstetrician to refer, and referral too late for diagnosis to be made during the first trimester.

7.1 Techniques

There are four main diagnostic methods, of which ultrasound scanning is the only one that is non-invasive. Chorionic villus sampling (CVS), amniocentesis and fetal blood sampling (cordocentesis) are invasive methods for obtaining a sample of fetal tissue for laboratory analysis. It is often necessary to use more than one procedure to obtain a definitive diagnosis; for instance CVS may be followed by confirmatory amniocentesis, and the detection of an abnormality by ultrasound scanning may lead to fetal blood sampling.

One of the most important considerations in prenatal diagnosis is its timing in relation to stage of pregnancy. Women prefer to have tests as early as possible and results as quickly as possible, but so far CVS is the only procedure that is reliable during the first trimester. Fortunately, chorionic villus material is suitable for DNA, biochemical and cytogenetic investigations, and, provided that they are counselled early enough in pregnancy, most couples at risk of a single-gene or chromosomal disorder can take advantage of this approach. Tests for congenital abnormalities and – in younger women – for risk of chromosomal disorders must still be done in the second trimester, but there is great research interest in developing methods that can be applied earlier.

Other extremely important considerations are the accuracy of the result, the safety of the sampling procedure and the time taken to obtain the result. Current information on these and other important aspects of the invasive procedures is summarized in Table 15.

Table 15
Methods of prenatal diagnosis using transabdominal sampling techniques

| Method | Success rate (%) | Weeks of gestation | Karyotyping | | Fetal loss rate (%) |
			Waiting time for results	Reliability	
Chorionic villus sampling	> 99	≥ 9	hours – 10 days	Very high	1
Amniocentesis	> 99	≥ 15	10-20 days	Very high	1
Cordocentensis	> 95	≥ 18	3-4 days	Very high	1-2

7.1.1 *Fetal anomaly scanning*

One of the most important obstetric applications of ultrasound scanning is for the detection of fetal abnormality, but only the grossest morphological abnormalities can be detected in this way. Scanning is most often offered to pregnant women for confirming intrauterine gestation, gestational age, and fetal viability and number.

A formal "fetal anomaly scan" to detect congenital abnormalities involves use of a check-list and takes 15-20 minutes. If the scan is done at around 19 weeks' gestation, when fetal organs are sufficiently developed for malformations to be visible, an expert in fetal medicine can detect over 90% of major malformations (*33*). Fetal anomaly scanning is generally offered to women belonging to recognized risk groups, e.g. those with diabetes, raised serum AFP level, twins, or a history of fetal abnormality or possible exposure to a known teratogen. However, most congenital abnormalities occur in "normal" pregnancies and, if they are to be detected, fetal anomaly scanning must be offered routinely to all pregnant women. Trained ultrasonographers can detect over 70% of major malformations by routine scanning, which is steadily becoming more widespread. When a fetal abnormality is suspected, it must be confirmed by an expert in fetal medicine to avoid the risk of misinterpretation of the image leading to failure to detect abnormalities, misdiagnosis of abnormalities, or even abortion[1] of a healthy fetus.

Chromosomal abnormality in the fetus increases the risk of malformation. The detection of an abnormality by ultrasound is therefore an indicator of the need to proceed to fetal blood sampling and rapid karyotyping; 15-30% of fetuses in which an abnormality is detected on scanning prove to be chromosomally abnormal. In addition, as equipment and experience improve, it is becoming apparent that characteristics such as the shape of the fetal head or cerebellum, the length of the femur or the thickness of the skin at the back of the neck may indicate fetal chromosomal abnormality.

---
[1] See note on p. 2.

Ultrasound scanning is an integral part of all invasive procedures for fetal sampling or fetal treatment. Regular monitoring and randomized studies have shown no deleterious effect of the usual levels of ultrasound exposure in pregnancy (*34*).

7.1.2 *Amniocentesis*

Amniotic fluid is usually obtained by transabdominal puncture at 15–16 weeks' gestation, 15–20 ml containing enough viable cells for successful culture; it takes about 2 weeks to obtain enough mitoses for chromosome studies. High-quality preparations are needed for detailed study by chromosome banding. A DNA diagnosis (using PCR) can often be done directly on amniotic fluid cells, but chorionic villus material is a better source of DNA.

There has long been uncertainty about the obstetric risk of amniocentesis. Satisfactory risk data are available only for amniocentesis done between 15 and 19 weeks. A modern, well-designed Danish study that compared risk between two randomly selected groups of women under 35 years of age showed a 1% increased risk of miscarriage in the amniocentesis group, and a slightly increased risk of respiratory distress of the newborn and of common mild, correctable, orthopaedic deformities such as club foot.

A number of investigators have recently begun to perform amniocentesis at between 11 and 15 weeks. Similar success rates in obtaining samples and karyotyping were found in a randomized comparison of amnio-centesis and CVS at 10–13 weeks (*35*). The procedure is the same as for amniocentesis in the second trimester but, as the amount of amniotic fluid removed represents a much greater proportion of the total, the effect on fetal viability, developmental mechanisms and lung function might be proportionately greater. Data on risk are difficult to evaluate because of the small numbers of subjects to date and the lack of controls. A randomized trial is needed to evaluate the safety and efficacy of early amniocentesis.

7.1.3 *Chorionic villus sampling*

Chorionic villus material can be obtained in the first trimester of pregnancy, using either a catheter passed through the uterine cervix or a needle inserted through the abdominal wall. The latter technique is possible at any stage of pregnancy, provided that the placenta is accessible. Many more fetal cells are obtained than with amniocentesis, allowing quick and simple DNA diagnostic methods to be used, although chromosome studies can be more complicated.

Rapid karyotyping may be performed on cytotrophoblastic cells either immediately after sampling or after 24–48 hours in culture. This allows reliable counts of chromosome number, but "direct" chromosome preparations are difficult to band and are unsuitable for detecting subtle chromosomal anomalies. High-quality preparations can be obtained by culturing the mesenchymal cells of the chorionic villi, but this takes 10–20 days. Fluorescent *in situ* hybridization (FISH) is a new method for detecting numerical chromosome abnormalities in non-dividing cells; it uses fluorescent DNA probes for specific sequences characteristic for different chromosomes and offers very considerable possibilities for increasing the range and accuracy of genetic diagnosis using chorionic villus material.

In a small percentage of cases, placental mosaicism can lead to a false-positive diagnosis of fetal abnormality. However, this does not cause major problems for experienced investigators.

Collaborative studies in Canada, Denmark and the USA of transcervical CVS have shown only a slight increase in fetal loss as compared with amniocentesis (*36*). The Danish study also included a comparison of transcervical and transabdominal CVS and showed that the total rate of fetal loss, including the effect of CVS itself, after transabdominal CVS was not significantly different from that following amniocentesis (6.4% vs 6.6%). By contrast, a randomized European study (*37*) showed a significant (4.6%) reduction in the chance of a live birth after CVS compared with that after amniocentesis. Data from the largest centre participating in the study (where all tests are done by two experienced clinicians) showed no excess loss rate for CVS as compared with amniocentesis; this result is consistent with the experience of the majority of experienced expert centres (*38*).

7.1.4 *Fetal blood sampling (cordocentesis)*

Fetal blood can be obtained safely only at or after 18 weeks of pregnancy. Sampling is by ultrasound-guided transabdominal needle puncture of the fetal cord insertion. When sampling is performed by a well-trained operator in the mid-second trimester, the average fetal loss rate is 1–2% (*39*). Fetal blood sampling was first used for prenatal diagnosis of blood disorders, but its commonest current application is for the rapid karyotyping of fetal lymphocytes when a major malformation has been detected by ultrasound.

7.1.5 *Fetal tissue biopsy*

Although advances in human genome mapping are likely to make most inherited diseases diagnosable by DNA analysis of chorionic tissue, it may still be necessary to obtain a sample of fetal skin, liver or muscle to diagnose some inherited diseases. Fetal tissue biopsy is best done at 19–20 weeks' gestation. Experience is still very limited, and the risks of the procedure are probably higher than for fetal blood sampling.

7.1.6 *New prenatal diagnostic techniques*

Clear-cut evidence of benefits, experimental evaluation of efficacy and –

as far as possible – of risks, and controlled trials are all needed before any new prenatal diagnostic technique is used in clinical practice.

7.2 Current research on fetal sampling

7.2.1 *Obtaining fetal cells from maternal blood*

The commonest reason for refusing prenatal diagnosis given by couples who would otherwise wish to know the diagnosis for their baby is the risk associated with invasive fetal sampling procedures. There is therefore considerable interest in developing risk-free methods of fetal sampling. The recovery and analysis of fetal cells from maternal peripheral blood may offer such a possibility.

Three types of fetal nucleated cells, namely lymphocytes, syncytio-trophoblast cells and erythroblasts, may be identified and isolated from maternal blood by exploiting antigenic differences between mother and fetus. The presence of fetal cells in maternal blood has often been verified by PCR techniques. It is generally agreed that, for success and accuracy, use of fetal cells must involve three major steps:

- identification of fetal cells by sensitive and highly specific monoclonal antibodies;
- an enrichment process (e.g. fluorescence-activated cell sorting), because so few fetal cells are present in maternal peripheral blood;
- genetic analysis of the collected cells by highly sensitive techniques such as FISH and PCR.

Of the three types of fetal cells found in the maternal circulation, erythroblasts seem to be the best candidates for prenatal testing. Fetal sex has been correctly identified in 94–100% of pregnancies at 8–19 weeks of gestation, and two cases of trisomy 21, one of trisomy 18 and one of Klinefelter syndrome have been detected by FISH for chromosome-specific DNA sequences, using sorted maternal blood (*40*). Many problems remain to be solved, such as how to deal with the almost inevitable maternal contamination, and the possible effects of ABO- or Rh-incompatibility on the survival of fetal red cells in the mother's circulation.

It is possible that the identification of fetal cells in maternal blood will provide a reliable non-invasive screening method for identifying fetuses at substantially increased risk of abnormality, so that the mother can then be offered a more invasive method for definitive diagnosis.

7.2.2 *Preimplantation genetic diagnosis*

Prenatal diagnosis is most distressing for couples at high genetic risk, as they suffer great anxiety in every pregnancy and may terminate two or three pregnancies[1] before having a healthy child. Such couples therefore

---

[1] See note on p. 2.

often ask for diagnosis before the embryo implants, in order to avoid the issue of abortion altogether. It is now possible to make a DNA diagnosis on a single cell. If DNA diagnosis is combined with *in vitro* fertilization (IVF) techniques, preimplantation diagnosis seems a realistic possibility. Several approaches are being considered for couples at risk of disorders with mendelian inheritance patterns.

Preimplantation genetic analysis requires easy access to gametes and embryos at the cleavage or blastocyst stage, and therefore to an IVF centre, efficient and safe microbiopsy procedures, and sensitive and specific techniques for analysis of the genetic material in one or a few cells. This is at present a very high-technology approach, subject to all the limitations of IVF.

Possible approaches include the removal and examination of the first polar body extruded from the unfertilized egg at ovulation, and embryo biopsy on the third day after fertilization (the 6–10 cell stage), when one or two cells may be removed for testing without any detrimental effect on the embryo. Several centres are already testing these methods in clinical practice. Indications have included risk of X-linked disorders (haemophilia and Lesch–Nyhan syndrome), and α-1-antitrypsin deficiency, Tay–Sachs disease and cystic fibrosis. Up to November 1993, total clinical experience consisted of 115 clinical cycles of stimulation of ovulation, resulting in 21 pregnancies and 13 births (rate per cycle: 11.0%). There were two misdiagnoses, one in sex determination on a single blastomere and one in testing a first polar body for cystic fibrosis by PCR.

Blastocyst biopsy is another possibility. Optimal culture media can greatly increase the proportion of fertilized eggs that develop *in vitro* to the blastocyst stage, and 10 cells or more may be removed for diagnosis from a blastocyst. This would increase the reliability of DNA analysis and permit two or more specimens to be run in parallel. However, no blastocysts have yet been transferred after biopsy.

7.3 Fetal therapy

Fetal disorders can be divided into four groups:

- anomalies that are fatal or untreatable and incompatible with prolonged life;
- anomalies that are best treated after delivery;
- anomalies that benefit from the mode and timing of delivery;
- anomalies that might benefit from prenatal treatment.

In utero fetal therapy is one of the goals of prenatal diagnosis. Fetal intraperitoneal blood transfusion for the treatment of severe rhesus haemolytic disease was pioneered in 1963. The modern method of treatment by umbilical cord infusion following direct needling under ultrasound guidance permits survival of up to 90% of affected fetuses (*41*). However, only a limited number of other congenital disorders

Table 16
Congenital disorders for which fetal therapy is available

Type of therapy	Disorder and treatment
Medical	• Use of dexamethasone in congenital adrenal hyperplasia (female fetuses only) • Use of vitamin B_{12} in certain types of methylmalonic acidaemia • Biotin supplementation in multiple carboxylase deficiency • Maternal folate supplementation for risk of neural tube defects • Cardiac medication in fetal arrhythmia • Maternal i.v. gammaglobulin administration in alloimmune thrombocytopenia
Intravasal	• Blood transfusion in fetal anaemia secondary to alloimmunization, virally mediated red blood cell aplasia, haemorrhage • Platelet transfusion in alloimmune thrombocytopenia
Surgery	• Open-uterus procedures (diaphragmatic hernia, urinary tract obstruction, sacrococcygeal teratoma) • Closed-uterus procedures (needle aspiration), placement of chronic shunts for cystic lesions of the chest or urinary tract obstruction
Gene therapy	• Haematopoietic stem-cell transplantation (haemoglobinopathies, severe combined immunodeficiency) • Germ-line gene therapy

benefit from *in utero* treatment at present (Table 16). Experimental, clinical and laboratory investigations are required to determine which procedures are sufficiently safe and effective for use in treating the human fetus.

Research on fetal therapy has a promising future. For example, recent progress in the postnatal therapy of leukaemia and severe combined immunodeficiency disease (SCID) by bone marrow transplantation (BMT) raises the possibility that this technique might be a useful form of replacement therapy for a variety of genetically determined disorders, including blood disorders, and more general metabolic errors. Problems with postnatal BMT include difficulties in finding an HLA-compatible donor, existing sequelae of the genetic defect, graft rejection, graft-versus-host disease and side-effects of preparatory immunosuppression. Some of these problems might be avoided by transplantation *in utero*: the fetus is immunotolerant up to about 20 weeks and would accept foreign grafts. Recently, successful engraftment has been reported in three human fetuses affected by bare lymphocyte syndrome, SCID and β-thalassaemia (*42*). However, there remains uncertainty about whether donor cell proliferation is sufficient to treat such diseases effectively and how long donor cells persist.

Figure 11
General structure of a comprehensive genetic service at national or regional level

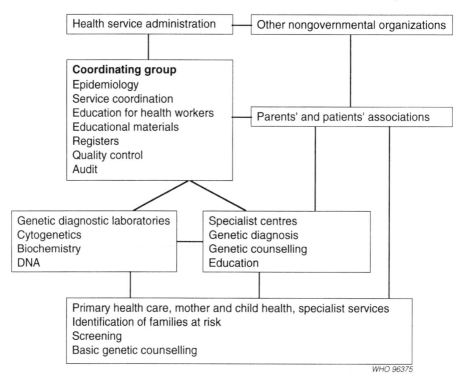

WHO 96375

7.4 **Conclusions**

Obstetricians are among the most important partners in the multidisciplinary collaboration that exists in modern medical genetics. Many approaches are now available within the framework of care during pregnancy to help women ensure that they have healthy babies. Prenatal diagnosis is an important option that should be available; it often provides reassurance, may contribute to optimal care for a fetus or neonate with a known disorder, and allow parents the option of terminating pregnancy.[1] Specialists in fetal medicine are now needed in all health care systems.

8. **Organization of genetic services**

In most countries of the world, genetic services are at an early stage of development or may be non-existent. Where medical genetics is a recognized specialty, however, there is now considerable interest in extending genetic services more widely, so that the community can benefit from progress in understanding the human genome.

---

[1] See note on p. 2.

Table 17
Specialities needed for a comprehensive genetic service

Family planning

Haematology

Health education

Medical genetics

Obstetrics

Oncology

Paediatrics

Paediatric pathology

Primary care

Public health

Public information resources

The general structure of a comprehensive genetic service including both specialist and community components is shown in Fig. 11. In a country with a fully developed service, there is likely to be a network of clinical genetic services and a national clinical genetics society; the clinical specialties listed in Table 17 will have an organized relationship with one another and easy mutual access. However, this degree of organization represents the end-point of a process of development, and many countries now have to consider how they can best move towards this optimal situation. A great deal of progress can be made by coordinating the services already available at the public health, secondary and primary care levels.

8.1 Basic public health services

The approaches listed on pages 34–35 are simple and inexpensive, and lead to large benefits in health. They should be integrated into health systems at all levels of development.

8.2 Genetics in secondary care

Where there are few or no clinical geneticists, the demand for genetic services is met, as far as possible, by other interested specialists. Paediatricians, for example, who diagnose the commoner congenital and hereditary disorders, do their best to inform the parents of the pattern of inheritance and risk of recurrence, and of the possibilities for prenatal diagnosis when appropriate. In the case of single-gene disorders, the parents' extended families should also be informed of their high risk and be offered testing and counselling. However, it can be difficult to take a genetic family history in a busy clinic, and hospital specialists are rarely in a position to pursue family studies, so that many individuals who could benefit from genetic counselling are missed. The possibility of referral to a clinical geneticist greatly improves both the range of diagnosis available and the delivery of genetic counselling to families.

Knowledge of the genetic element in many other fields of medicine is rapidly increasing, and cytogenetic, biochemical and DNA diagnostic laboratories are needed to provide services for specialists such as paediatricians, cardiologists, haematologists and oncologists. Once the importance of a genetic service is recognized, such existing elements can be coordinated so as to develop the service further. In addition, parents' and patients' support groups for locally important conditions may already exist and can be recruited to support service development.

There is evidence that patients live longer and enjoy a better quality of life if they attend a specialist treatment centre, rather than being treated within the general paediatric service. Affected families benefit from contact with each other and with a support group. Specialist treatment centres can also be a focus for the development of a disease-oriented genetic service, e.g. for neural tube defects or haemoglobin disorders. The skills and infrastructure needed for services of this type are similar to those required for all genetic services. Once established, a disease-oriented service can evolve into a broader genetic service, as has already happened in various places, including Cyprus and Sardinia.

8.3 Genetics in primary health care

A genetic service needs a base in primary health care, both because families at high risk can be counselled only if they are recognized and referred, and because of the increasing role of genetic population screening. At present, even where genetic services are widely available, access is limited by lack of awareness, screening and counselling at the primary care level (6). Primary care workers should:

- be able to give correct information on genetic risks that are common locally and on ways to reduce them;
- be aware of common genetic disorders and their management;
- be aware of local specialist centres, and refer affected children and couples at risk appropriately;
- be able to take a genetic family history so as to identify people in need of referral to specialist services;
- arrange screening and provide counselling for carriers of single-gene disorders, inform relatives of the high chance of their also being carriers (50% for siblings) and offer them testing;
- give advice on reducing the risk of common disorders with genetic predisposition;
- understand the basic ethical principles and techniques of genetic counselling.

At the primary care level, genetic advice needs to be seen as an integral component of the service "packages" that should be delivered to people in specific clinical situations.

8.4 Education and information

8.4.1 *Education for health workers*

Efforts should be made in countries at all levels of development to improve awareness of genetics among health care professionals, ways in which new genetic knowledge can be applied and the resources available locally. Medical genetics should therefore be included in medical, nursing and midwifery teaching curricula, which should also cover special genetic issues of particular interest to the local population, e.g. screening for haemoglobin disorders and counselling with respect to consanguineous marriage. Refresher courses that include training in genetic counselling techniques should also be organized for health workers already in practice, few of whom have received any training in this area.

8.4.2 *Information for patients and families*

People with a specific disorder, and their families, require full and clear information, particularly if the disorder is rare or if they do not have access to a specialist service. Support groups provide many excellent information materials that are helpful to health workers as well as families. However, these materials naturally tend to be disease-oriented, and are not primarily concerned with screening.

8.4.3 *Information in schools*

The teaching of human genetics in a simple and appropriate manner should be incorporated into school curricula at a stage when it will reach every child. A knowledge of the recessive mode of inheritance is probably the most important part of such teaching since it helps people to understand the transmission of cystic fibrosis and the haemoglobin disorders. Teaching that anyone can be the carrier of an inherited disease also helps to prevent prejudice and misinformation.

8.4.4 *Information for the media*

Professionals in genetics, health education and the media can work together to increase the awareness of genetics among the adult population. Suitable media include television documentaries on specific diseases, stories containing a character with a genetic disease and accurate newspaper accounts of advances in genetics. If good information materials are available for patients and families, they will also be available to the media and can help to increase accuracy of reporting.

8.5 Information materials

Experience has shown the need for specific educational materials at each stage in a screening programme. As already mentioned, counsellors can save a great deal of time by giving people at risk of common disorders informative leaflets to read and keep for future reference, or videos to watch, before counselling. The following points should also be noted:

- Pregnant women require a comprehensive but simple outline of the genetic services provided in the course of antenatal care. Examples of materials that provide this are the WHO documents on haemoglobinopathies.[1]
- Extremely simple information is needed before services such as screening for carrier status for recessively inherited disorders are offered.
- When a genetic risk is identified, there is a need for comprehensive and clear information, specific to the individual or the couple concerned. In view of the great diversity of genetic risks, this can be a major challenge.
- When prenatal diagnosis is under discussion, the woman or couple will require comprehensive written and oral information on the implications of the test, the risks to the pregnancy, the accuracy of the results and possible methods for the termination of the pregnancy.[2]

Little high-quality health education material on these topics is available in most countries. This problem could be solved relatively economically as models of such materials need to be prepared only once (preferably in collaboration with an expert in health education), after which they can made available nationally and internationally and adapted for local use with suitable modifications.

In practice, providing genetic screening and giving carriers good information materials is an effective way of informing a wider population, because people will discuss these matters with family and friends. Good information materials for patients are also useful for doctors and nurses, who should be sent copies of the materials given to their patients.

8.6 Role of patients' and parents' support groups

Support groups play an essential role in the development of genetic services. In developing countries, the first effective step towards establishing a control programme for haemoglobin disorders is often the formation of a support group (7).

Support groups provide psychological support for families by bringing them into contact with others with a similar problem. All families with an affected member, and carriers of specific genetic disorders, should be put in touch with relevant support groups where those exist. Such groups identify the concerns of families and allow the community to participate in developing services. They draw attention to gaps in service provision and in research, and provide help by means such as raising funds for research

---

[1] Modell B. *Educational materials on haemoglobinopathies: alpha thalassaemia.*
Modell B. *Educational materials on haemoglobinopathies: beta thalassaemia.*
Geneva, World Health Organization, 1994 (unpublished documents WHO/HDP/EM/HB.BT/94.4 and WHO/HDP/EM/HB.AT/94.5, obtainable on request from Human Genetics, World Health Organization, 1211 Geneva 27, Switzerland).
[2] See note on p. 2.

perceived as relevant by patients and families. They support public health activities such as screening, and help in informing and educating both the public and health professionals. Screening seems to increase public support for such groups and concern for patients; carriers will often feel that, as they share an important genetic trait, they "join a family".

Input from support groups increases the sensitivity of doctors to the concerns of those affected by genetic disorders, and can also help patients to resist external pressures to either accept or reject prenatal diagnosis. Their involvement in comprehensive control programmes provides public reassurance that the patients' interests are being safeguarded.

8.7 Developing genetic services

The relative roles of government and private health services, the available resources, the pattern of use of such resources, and the nature of the primary health care infrastructure are all aspects of the health care system that affect strategies for providing genetic diagnosis and counselling. In some countries, the government provides basic services only; more sophisticated services are very limited or available only in the private sector. Specialist services (public or private) are then likely to develop in response to obvious need, so that at least some families obtain access to diagnosis, treatment and counselling.

In the absence of organized primary health care, it may be impossible to provide genetic population screening. Screening tests will then be carried out by individual clinicians (e.g. private obstetricians), but the number of people who benefit from such tests will be relatively small. The health care infrastructure *per se*, rather than the amount of money spent on health care, is the main determinant of the feasibility of community-based services. In the USA, for example, in the absence of a primary health care infrastructure, specially trained genetic counsellors are needed, while in the United Kingdom it seems possible that basic genetic counselling may be integrated into the primary health care services provided by general (family) practitioners.

Where a primary health care infrastructure is well developed, genetic screening is feasible and indeed likely to become necessary.

8.8 Audit of services

Programmes are being developed in several countries to monitor the effects of prevention services for genetic disorders, in order to identify and correct shortcomings. These programmes depend to a large extent on the use of registers; cancer registries, for example, can be used to monitor the number of new cases of familial cancer syndromes. Patients can then be followed up through their case notes to assess the extent to which genetic aspects have been taken into account and to evaluate the amount and quality of the genetic information provided to other family members. With the help of registers, prenatal diagnosis services can be

Figure 12

Example of the use of a patient register for the audit of treatment and prevention

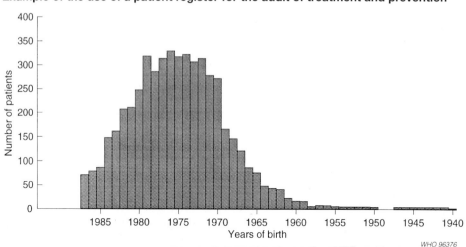

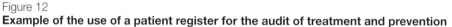

WHO 96376

The data are taken from the Italian register of thalassaemic patients. The chart shows relatively few patients more than 25 years old, not because they die before the age of 25 but because modern management was introduced in Italy about 25 years previously. Most severely affected children born before that time died in infancy. When a register is regularly updated, the movement of the "leading edge" of the curve towards the right is a measure of the continuing survival of older patients. Confidential enquiry into causes of death can be used to measure success in treatment. Similarly, the "trailing edge" of the curve shows a decreasing number of new patients born each year as a result of genetic counselling and the use of prenatal diagnosis. Since the uptake of prenatal diagnosis for thalassaemia in Italy is nearly 100%, the fall in the thalassaemia major birth rate is a measure of the effectiveness of efforts to inform, and provide screening and counselling to, the whole population.

assessed by means of relatively simple criteria, such as the birth-rate of affected individuals, the choices that couples at risk make with respect to using prenatal diagnosis, the numbers of prenatal diagnoses performed, and the numbers of births of children with avoidable conditions. Such assessment also makes it possible to evaluate the role of informed choice by the parents. The use of a patient register in the audit of treatment and prevention is illustrated in Fig. 12.

8.9 Conclusions

In almost all countries, greater attention should now be paid to the development and coordination of genetic services. Community genetic services are relatively inexpensive and, set against the great social and financial burden of chronic disease, highly cost-effective. One of the main problems in delivering genetic services appears to be the difficulty of informing both the health professions and the community of the real significance of genetic problems.

It is relatively inexpensive to bring key elements together to form a management group at the national, regional or district level, which can then collaborate with the health authorities to develop genetic services. The activities of the group will depend on the local level of service development, but the concept of the service will often need to be developed from scratch. It is important to ensure that there are no unnecessary boundaries between the disciplines involved in delivering genetic services to the population. Continuing professional education and re-education are needed.

9. Ethical, social and legal aspects of genetic technology in medicine

Popular perceptions of human genetics are varied, tinged with metaphor and myth, and subject to polemics. The metaphors are largely the scientists' own: some refer to the Human Genome Project as "The Book of Man" or the "New Holy Grail" (43). There is public uncertainty as to whether the Project is the final "slippery slope", the ultimate form of "playing God" or of "interfering with Nature" (44). Public concerns reflect a certain disillusion with science and technology, which are now seen as not working solely for the benefit of humanity, and a perception of the failure of governments to provide adequately for the disabled; there is also scepticism about priorities in government funding. In reality, the Human Genome Project does not raise any new problems but contains, and magnifies the complexity of, many basic ethical, legal and social issues. This section focuses on those issues as they relate to the proper use of genetic technology, rather than to the technology itself.

Genetic information has personal, familial and social implications. From an ethical, social and legal viewpoint, the important aspects of genetic testing include its largely predictive nature and the fact that a genetic diagnosis in one individual inevitably has implications for other family members. However, clinical geneticists have been testing and counselling affected families for many years without arousing major public concern. The growth in public interest is the consequence of the increasing ability to detect genetic risk in the absence of affected relatives, and the associated developments in genetic population screening. The public is right to be concerned because these developments, together with any associated errors or abuses, affect every member of society.

9.1 Genetic population screening

Genetic population screening can take the form of newborn screening, carrier screening or prenatal screening.

Newborn screening for treatable conditions is universally accepted as a routine part of neonatal care and, in most countries, the written consent of the parents is not required. An international ethics survey has identified newborn screening as the one area of genetic testing where participation should be mandatory, because it is in the interest of the at-risk child to be found, diagnosed and treated (45). Patients should be informed of such programmes; if they do not consent to neonatal screening, appropriate legal action can be taken in the name of the child.

Carrier screening involves the voluntary testing of asymptomatic young adults; it is accompanied by reproductive counselling. The birth of an affected child is no longer the entry point for genetic services in screened populations. Carrier screening is often offered to ethnically distinct populations and therefore raises the possibility of stigmatization. With the discovery of the cystic fibrosis gene, carrier screening is rapidly expanding. This reduces the risk of ethnic stigmatization on the one hand, but increases the risk of discrimination in insurance and employment on the other, since the status of "carrier" is commonly misunderstood and equated with presence of the disease. Informed consent and counselling are essential elements of carrier screening programmes (46).

Similarly, patients' consent should be obtained for any use of genetic samples for research purposes. In return, those involved in such research have the reciprocal obligation of providing information, choice and control regarding the use of DNA samples and the genetic information that they contain. In this way, public trust and participation will not be undermined or abused.

Prenatal screening is used, for example, in pregnant women of relatively advanced age. As diagnostic techniques become more sophisticated (e.g. ultrasound), or are offered earlier in time (e.g. CVS), the psychosocial impact of late abortions[1] may be reduced. At the same time, however, prenatal diagnosis can also be used for an increasing number of disorders, not all of which are necessarily serious or of immediate onset. The principle of freedom of choice should be maintained, but choice must be informed. The public therefore needs to be made more aware of the implications of genetic disorders (25).

9.2 Predictive genetic testing

For many later-onset genetic disorders, diagnosis no longer depends on the first appearance of symptoms. Young adults, children, the fetus and even the embryo can now be tested presymptomatically for the presence of genes that may not be expressed until much later in life (e.g. Huntington disease) or that very are variable in expression (e.g. myotonic dystrophy).

Autonomy and non-directive counselling have long been the hallmarks of genetic testing. Individual choices are influenced by personal values with regard to the sancity of human life, the wish to avoid human suffering, cultural attitudes, and the socioeconomic consequences of the absence of

---

[1] See note on p. 2.

treatment or of adequate support for the disabled or chronically ill. The problem then arises, however, as to who should decide on the acceptability of, for example, preimplantation testing or abortion[1] for a condition that will not become manifest for decades or that may be relatively mild. Traditionally, abortion[1] was acceptable – and often legally permissible – when there was a "high risk of a severe genetic disorder", but this view was taken at a time when only a few conditions could be detected prenatally. However, there are at present no clear grounds for changing this criterion. Recording and reporting the choices actually made by informed people provides a simple mechanism for observing how people use genetic information in practice (6).

Predictive testing can also be used for non-genetic reasons; in some countries, amniocentesis and CVS have been used for prenatal sex selection of male children. Genetic technology should not be used for such purposes.

9.3 Detecting susceptibility genes

A "susceptibility gene" is a gene whose presence increases the risk of an individual's developing a multifactorial disorder (e.g. cancer, heart disease). For any such disorder to occur, however, additional environmental factors such as inappropriate diet or lifestyle, and perhaps other predisposing genes, may be required. There is thus a sliding scale from clear-cut "carrier" status, via "predictive" status, to "susceptibility" status. Because susceptibility information tends to be provided in terms of risk factors and probabilities, that is, expressed in percentages or as relative risks, the likelihood of misunderstanding and therefore of discrimination is increased. It remains to be seen whether susceptibility information can simply be factored into classical insurance and pre-employment selection, or whether safeguards are necessary to avoid the information being used to the disadvantage of people at risk.

The principle of solidarity (i.e. of risk-sharing and risk-spreading in society) argues for equitable access to services such as insurance and to employment (47). Voluntary, individual participation in susceptibility testing in order to try to influence the timing and severity of possible eventual manifestations of disorder should not lead to economic loss, nor should such testing be imposed by the state in order to reduce the costs of long-term medical care. Moreover, the aim of encouraging individual responsibility for health would be undermined if such information were not kept confidential.

9.4 Is there a right not to be informed?

Apart from neonatal screening for metabolic conditions that require immediate treatment, genetic testing must be voluntary (46). Because of

---

[1] See note on p. 2.

their right to inviolability and privacy, people should not be tested against their will or given information that they do not wish to have. Nevertheless, genetic information also has social and family implications. For example, testing could be associated with obtaining certain services or benefits (in the same way that school entry may be linked to immunization status) or with access to particular civil status (in Cyprus, for example, thalassaemia testing is required before marriage). If it is decided that a particular genetic test is in the public interest, and legislation has been adopted that makes it compulsory, the individual is obliged to find out his or her genetic status. However, it remains an open question whether people can be forced to know their genetic status in the absence of any such overriding public interest (*48*).

The familial nature of genetic information creates special obligations that extend beyond the patient. While an individual may wish to remain uninformed, the same degree of freedom may not apply in intraconjugal or intrafamilial decision-making, e.g. with regard to reproduction. The principle of mutuality within families carries certain *moral* obligations which might operate against the creation of new *legal* obligations that could be harmful to marital and family relationships. A future partner or a relative may well have a greater moral claim on genetic information for use in making reproductive choices than third parties have for other purposes. Under current legal constructs in certain countries, deliberate and conscious failure to know, or failure to warn, may be legally actionable between family members, as it is against physicians (*49*).

A right not to know is distinct from a right not to be tested. It could be argued that the full realization of the "right not to know" (if it exists at all) is possible only if the person concerned is knowledgeable about genetic risk, about the feasibility of testing and about the implications of the results, so as to be able to make a really "informed" choice not to know.

Finally, although testing for the benefit of other family members is always subject to individual consent, this can be problematic when DNA samples are needed from young children, who cannot consent. Children are individuals, but also family members and members of society. Genetic testing of children to help others make informed reproductive decisions is an issue that requires further study.

9.5 Human rights and duties

Respect for human dignity is the source of all human rights and duties. While the formulation of such rights and duties in the genetic arena is in its infancy, increased possibilities for genetic testing and information bring some of them to the forefront. Of these, the right to privacy is crucial.

The sophisticated technology available for information handling and in the field of genetics inevitably creates concern that a highly intimate personal issue – genetic decision-making – will be subject to scrutiny. The very notion of privacy has undergone a metamorphosis, its focus shifting from control over personal property to control over information about the individual (50). In human genetics, privacy is closely tied to the right to liberty, especially as concerns reproductive choice. What is often forgotten, however, is that liberty in research is itself a fundamental right, as is that of the citizen to benefit from such research. Failure to offer equitable access to genetic services is a failure to respect the rights of all citizens equally.

9.6 Data protection

The proliferation of genetic information requires a heightened awareness of the need for data protection; in fact, the protection of medical information in general needs to be strengthened and affirmed (46). Much genetic information (e.g. on blood group or HLA type) is used in routine medical practice and could be described as "value-neutral". However, information related to disease susceptibility is sometimes highly sensitive, especially when treatment is not available, and could attract the stigmatization usually associated with disability. In the absence of proper public education and understanding of genetic conditions, such information should be coded and subject to individual consent before it is released to third parties. The data should be included in collaborative or international research only when anonymity can be assured.

The free circulation of coded genetic data is essential if progress is to be made in genetic research and development of improved treatment. In this respect, the patenting of anonymous sequences of the human genome (that is, sequences without known function) (51) is detrimental to international collaboration and the sharing of research results, which depend on the open and free circulation of information among scientists. Traditionally, valid patent claims for specified innovative uses can be distinguished from such broad ownership claims (51). Similarly, financial rewards for obtaining DNA samples or genetic information run contrary to the principle of the non-commercialization of the human individual.

9.7 Genetic counselling

If the objective of medical genetic services is "to help people with a genetic disadvantage to live and to reproduce as normally as possible" (3, 12) by identifying people at risk and allowing them an informed choice among the options available, its realization depends on counselling. Counselling should be considered a condition *sine qua non* for any genetic testing.

Counselling helps both affected and unaffected people to enjoy more fulfilling lives and to safeguard their own and their family's health. In this approach, patient care and reproductive choice are complementary rather than competing aspects of the control of genetic disorders. As previously mentioned, genetic counselling requires accurate genetic knowledge, the ability to communicate, and time. It cannot be undertaken without training and adequate supervision or without proper compensation under state health or private insurance schemes. Contact with relatives should be through the consulting family member(s); when the relatives are themselves at high risk for a serious disorder, however, different considerations may apply (25).

Other ethical issues in genetic counselling are discussed in section 6.3.

9.8 Consensus ethics

In 1989, an international survey of ethics in the practice of human genetics revealed several areas of consensus (although there may well be cultural differences in the translation of this consensus into practice). The principles of accessibility, autonomy, non-directive counselling, consent and choice, and respect for confidentiality and the integrity of the individual are widely accepted (29). The efforts of the Council of Europe to draw up a bioethics convention, as well as UNESCO's work on the development of an international instrument for the protection of the human genome, represent steps to uphold these principles. It is strongly recommended that international, regional and national instruments should affirm these areas of consensus in medical genetics and research.

9.9 Autonomous decision-making versus regulation in society

Bioethics and much associated legislation is largely concerned with conflicts of rights. The adoption of an adversarial approach to human genetics would be extremely detrimental to the well-being of affected persons, their families and the communities concerned. This is especially important because of the personal, familial and social nature of genetic disease and genetic information, and because genetic reproductive decision-making affects not only current relationships but also future generations. Individual, professional and collective responsibility for decision-making should be based on public education and widespread access to precise genetic information, not on an adversarial approach or on claims of rights.

Public discussion, education and participation in choosing the direction of research, in the development of public health programmes and in decisions on priorities and funding are essential. Any regulation should be limited to those areas reflecting an informed public consensus.

9.10 Conclusions

The broadest ethical issue in the area of genetic services is their limited availability. Recent dramatic advances in the development of DNA techniques and their possible medical application make it necessary to update strategies for the control of genetic diseases. Progress in genetic testing techniques, which is much more rapid than progress in treatment, raises social and ethical issues concerned not with the technology itself but with its proper use. In this regard, it is of the utmost importance that scientific, medical and lay organizations should ensure that information and technology are used to preserve the dignity of the individual. The misuse of information can be avoided through discussions at different levels (health care professionals, policy-makers, mass media, schools, etc.) in order to establish a firm understanding of the actual and potential applications of new genetic technology and the achievements of human genome research.

10. Conclusions and recommendations

The Scientific Group emphasized that the remarkable advances in international human genome research and molecular biology would dramatically increase both the potential and the requirement for genetic approaches to the prevention and treatment of a wide spectrum of diseases. The Group summarized its recommendations and conclusions as follows:

1. Genetic approaches for health improvement should be fully integrated into general health services and should reflect the objectives of socioeconomic development.

2. In almost all countries additional attention should now be paid to the development and coordination of genetic services. This should involve the identification and · organization of existing resources, collection of accurate epidemiological data, education of health professionals, ensuring the implementation of the recommended public health approaches, training of specialists in clinical genetics, ensuring the availability of laboratory diagnostic services (especially karyotyping and DNA analysis), and developing appropriate health education materials for the public.

3. Developing countries, where the frequency of genetic disorders is particularly high, should be encouraged to set up training centres for clinical and laboratory diagnosis and the management of genetic disorders. These centres should form an integral part of the general health services.

4. International collaboration should be encouraged, with the aim of improving genetic health education at all levels, particularly through the development of appropriate educational aids.

5. Genetic screening should not be imposed on an uninformed public, and means should therefore be found to improve the community's understanding of human heredity.

6. Screening of newborn infants for treatable conditions should become a routine practice and should be recommended in the interests of all children.

7. Prenatal diagnosis is an important option that should be available to women. Specialists in fetal medicine are now needed in nearly all countries.

8. Information on the increased risk of chromosomal disorders and miscarriage with advancing maternal age should form an integral part of family planning and other health programmes for women.

9. To prevent congenital disorders, early (prereproductive) immunization against rubella is recommended, and the prevention of rhesus haemolytic disease by appropriate screening and administration of anti-D globulin after delivery should be further developed.

10. Families with premature onset of common conditions such as coronary heart disease, diabetes, stroke and cancer should be identified; advice on lifestyle should be provided and surveillance arranged when appropriate.

11. In order to make the best use of available resources, primary health care workers should be trained in taking genetic family histories and in providing basic advice; specialist centres would then be better able to deal with the patients referred for more complex management.

12. The result of human genome research should be applied internationally for the control of genetic disorders and of other major health problems in which there is a genetic predisposition.

13. National and international bodies should collaborate to ensure that genetic markers (and information defining them) are freely available to all countries for the study of familial and multifactorial disease. WHO could assist by recognizing a centre, or group of centres, that would work to ensure that gene markers, data and technology can be transferred quickly from developed to developing countries.

14. Advances in medical genetics should not be abused for non-medical purposes. The consent of the individual should be obtained for the use of DNA for research purposes.

15. The implications for genetic diagnosis and therapy of the patenting and ownership of DNA sequences, and of DNA technologies, are causing widespread concern; international agreement may be required to ensure that access to genetic technology, including gene therapy, is not restricted. Anonymous DNA sequences should not be the subject of patent protection.

16. Genetic information should be kept confidential, coded where possible, and subject to individual consent before release. Such information should not be used to the economic or social disadvantage of persons at risk.

17. The principles of accessibility, autonomy, non-directive counselling, consent, choice, confidentiality and respect for the integrity of the person should be universally applied to genetic counselling.

18. Information and educational materials about the health implications of the Human Genome Project should be made widely available in forms that can be freely used and copied.

19. WHO should contribute as appropriate to the dissemination of information on medical genetics and on associated ethical, legal and social issues.

Acknowledgements

The Scientific Group wishes to acknowledge the valuable contributions made to its discussions by Dr A.M. Kuliev, Research Reproductive Genetics Institute, Chicago, IL, USA (representing the WHO Regional Office of the Americas); and by the following WHO staff members: Mr S.S. Fluss, Chief, Health Legislation, Dr I. Gyarfas, Chief, Cardiovascular Diseases, Dr H. King, Diabetes and other Noncommunicable Diseases, Dr P.M. Shah, Child Health and Development.

References

1. McKusick VA. *Mendelian inheritance in man*, 10th ed. Baltimore, MD, Johns Hopkins University Press, 1994.

2. Forfar JO. Demography, vital statistics and the pattern of disease in childhood. In: Campbell AGM, McIntosh N, eds. *Forfar and Arniel's textbook of paediatrics*, 4th ed. Edinburgh, Churchill Livingstone, 1992.

3. *Community approaches to the control of hereditary diseases. Report of a WHO Advisory Group on Hereditary Diseases*. Geneva, World Health Organization, 1985 (unpublished document HMG/WG/85.10, available on request from Human Genetics, World Health Organization, 1211 Geneva 27, Switzerland).

4. Baird PA et al. Genetic disorders in children and young adults: a population study. *American journal of human genetics*, 1988, **42**:677–693.

5. Czeizel A, Sankaranarayanan K. The load of genetic and partly genetic disorders in man. 1. Congenital anomalies: estimates of detriment in terms of years of life lost and years of impaired life. *Mutation research*, 1984, **128**: 73–103.

6. Modell B, Kuliev AM, Wagner M. *Community genetics services in Europe*. Copenhagen, World Health Organization, Regional Office for Europe, 1992 (WHO Regional Publication, European Series No. 38).

7. *Prevention and control of haemoglobinopathies. Report of a Joint WHO/Thalassaemia International Federation Meeting and 7th Meeting of the WHO Working Group on the Control of Hereditary Anaemias*. Geneva, World Health Organization, 1993 (unpublished document WHO/HDP/TIF/HA/93.1, available on request from Human Genetics, World Health Organization, 1211 Geneva 27, Switzerland).

8. Glucose-6-phosphate dehydrogenase deficiency. Report of a WHO Working Group. *Bulletin of the World Health Organization* 1989, **67**:601–611.

9. *Guidelines for the control of haemoglobin disorders*. Geneva, World Health Organization, 1994 (unpublished document WHO/HDP/HB/GL/94.1, available on request from Human Genetics, World Health Organization, 1211 Geneva 27, Switzerland).

10. Bittles AH. *Consanguineous marriage: current global incidence and its relevance to demographic research*. Detroit, MI, Population Studies Center, University of Michigan, 1990 (Research Report No. 90-186).

11. Costa T, Scriver C, Childs B. The effect of Mendelian disease on human health: a measurement. *American journal of medical genetics*, 1985, **21**:231-242.

12. *Advances in diagnosis, treatment and prevention of hereditary diseases. Report of a World Health Organization meeting*. Geneva, World Health Organization, 1989 (unpublished document WHO/HDP/ADV/89.3, available on request from Human Genetics, World Health Organization, 1211 Geneva 27, Switzerland).

13. Czeizel A, Intody Z, Modell B. What proportion of congenital anomalies can be prevented? *British medical journal*, 1993, **306**:499-502.

14. de la Mata I et al. Incidence of congenital rubella syndrome in 19 regions of Europe in 1980-1986. *European journal of epidemiology*, 1989, **5**:106-109.

15. MRC Vitamin Research Group. Prevention of neural tube defects: results of the Medical Research Council vitamin study. *Lancet*, 1991, **338**:131-137.

16. Varekamp I et al. Carrier testing and prenatal diagnosis for hemophilia: experiences and attitudes of 549 potential and obligate carriers. *American journal of medical genetics*, 1990, **37**:147-154.

17. Cuckle HS, Wald NJ. Principles of screening. In: NJ Wald, ed. *Antenatal and neonatal screening*. Oxford, Oxford University Press, 1984.

18. Kaback M et al. Tay-Sachs disease – carrier screening, prenatal diagnosis, and the molecular era. An international perspective 1970-1993. *Journal of the American Medical Association,* 1993, **270**:2307-2315.

19. Stone MH et al. Comparison of audible sound transmission with ultrasound in screening for congenital dislocation of the hip. *I ancet*, 1990, **336**:421-422.

20. Illig R et al. Mental development in congenital hypothyroidism after neonatal screening. *Archives of disease in childhood*, 1987, **62**:1050-1055.

21. Neonatal screening for sickle cell disease. *Paediatrics*, 1989, 83 (Suppl.).

22. Balnaves ME et al. The impact of newborn screening on cystic fibrosis testing in Victoria, Australia. *Journal of medical genetics*, 1995, **32**:537-542.

23. Smith RA et al. Screening for Duchenne muscular dystrophy. *Archives of disease in childhood*, 1989, **64**:1017-1021.

24. Wald NJ et al. Antenatal maternal serum screening for Down's syndrome: results of a demonstration study. *British medical journal*, 1992, **305**:391-393.

25. Canadian Royal Commission on New Reproductive Technologies. *Proceed with care. Final report of the Canadian Royal Commission on New Reproductive Technologies, Vol. 2*. Ottawa, Canada Communications Group – Publishing, 1993.

26. **Czeizel AE.** Prevention of congenital abnormalities by periconceptional multivitamin supplementation. *British medical journal*, 1993, **306**:1645-8.

27. **Craufurd D et al.** Uptake of presymptomatic predictive testing for Huntington's disease. *Lancet*, 1989, ii:603-605.

28. **Sangani B et al.** Thalassaemia in Bombay: the role of medical genetics in developing countries. *Bulletin of the World Health Organization*, 1990, **68**:75-81.

29. **Fletcher JC, Berg K, Tranoy KE.** Ethical aspects of medical genetics. A proposal for guidelines in genetic counselling, prenatal diagnosis and screening. *Clinical genetics,* 1985, **27**:199-205.

30. **Weaver DD.** *Catalogue of prenatally diagnosed conditions*, 2nd ed. Baltimore, MD, Johns Hopkins University Press, 1992.

31. **Tului L, Brambati B.** Acceptance of first trimester prenatal diagnosis: analysis of the religious and socio-cultural characteristics. *Rivista di ostetrica, ginecologia pratica e medicina perinatale*, 1990, **5**:129-137.

32. **Milunsky A.** *Genetic disorders and the fetus*, 3rd ed. Baltimore, MD Johns Hopkins University Press, 1992.

33. **Luck CA.** Value of routine ultrasound scanning at 19 weeks: a four-year study of 8849 deliveries. *British medical journal*, 1992, **304**:1474-1476.

34. **Ewigman B, LeFevre M, Hesser J.** A randomised trial of routine prenatal ultrasound. *Obstetrics and gynaecology*, 1990, **76**:189-194.

35. **Byrne D et al.** Randomized study of early amniocentesis versus chorionic villus sampling: a technical and cytogenetic comparison of 650 patients. *Ultrasound obstetrics and gynecology*, 1991, **1**:235-240.

36. **Canadian Collaborative CVS-Amniocentesis Clinical Trial Group.** Multicentre randomised clinical trial of chorion villus sampling and amniocentesis. First report. *Lancet*, 1989, i:1-6.

37. **Medical Research Council Working Party on the Evaluation of Chorion Villus Sampling.** Medical Research Council European trial of chorion villus sampling. *Lancet*, 1991, **337**:1491-1499.

38. **Firth HV et al.** Severe limb abnormalities after chorion villus sampling at 56-66 days' gestation. *Lancet*, 1991, **337**:762-763.

39. **Romero R, Ghidini A, Santolaya J.** Fetal blood sampling. In: Milunsky A, ed. *Genetic disorders and the fetus*, 3rd ed. Baltimore, MD, Johns Hopkins University Press, 1992:649-682.

40. **Bianchi DW et al.** Erythroid-specific antibodies enhance detection of fetal nucleated erythrocytes in maternal blood. *Prenatal diagnosis*, 1993, **13**:293-300.

41. **American College of Obstetricians and Gynecologists.** Management of isoimmunization in pregnancy. *Technical bulletin*, 1990, **148**:1-6.

42. **Touraine JL et al.** In utero transplantation of hemopoietic stem cells in humans. *Transplantation proceedings*, 1991, **23**:1706-1708.

43. **Lewontin RC.** The dream of the human genome. *New York Times review*, 1992, 28:31-40.

44. **Nolan K, Swenson S.** New tools, new dilemmas: genetic frontiers. *Hastings Center report*, 1988, **18**:40-46.

45. Knoppers BM. Newborn screening and informed consent. In: Farriaux JP, Dhont JL, eds. *Proceedings of the 9th International Symposium on Neonatal Screening, Lille, France*. Amsterdam, Elsevier Excerpta Medica, 1994:15-24.

46. Knoppers BM, Chadwick R. The Human Genome Project: under an international legal and ethical microscope. *Science*, 1994, **265**:2033-2034.

47. Committee of the Health Council of the Netherlands. *Heredity: science and society*. The Hague, Health Council of the Netherlands, 1989.

48. Kielstein R, Sass H-M. Right not to know or duty to know? Prenatal screening for polycystic renal disease. *Journal of medical philosophy*, 1992, **17**:395-405.

49. Andrews LB. The double helix. *Houston law review*, 1992, 29(1):149-184.

50. *R.* v. *Dyment,* 2 SCR 417-442, 1988; Privacy Commissioner of Canada, Genetic Testing and Privacy, Minister of Supply and Services, 1992.

51. Eisenberg RS. Patenting the human genome. *Emory law journal*, 1990, **39**: 721-745.

World Health Organization Technical Report Series

---

* Prices in developing countries are 70% of those listed here.